MR.TEASEL
My Hero

MR. TEASEL
My Hero

by Jim Lindl

With Voices From The Wilderness

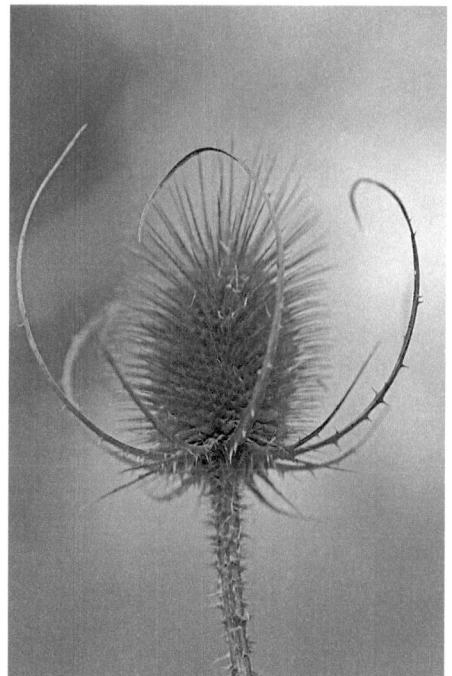

Wild Teasel Seed Pod

This beautiful spiny Teasel, and the following two individuals, along with their strength, wisdom and compassion, helped me lift unknown forces that were crushing my soul.

Dr. David Halverstadt D.C.
Dr. Wolf-Dieter Storl (Medical Anthropologist)

Copyright

MR.TEASEL My Hero

Copyright © 2016 by James R. (Jim) Lindl.

All Rights Reserved. No part of this book, including text and photographs, may be reproduced or transmitted in any form, by any electronic or mechanical means, including information storage and retrieval systems, without written permission from the publisher.

Book Design & Photographs © 2016 by Martha Lindl,
All Rights Reserved.

Book Cover: Wild Teasel On Background Texture © 2016,
All Rights Reserved.
Wild Teasel Image © 2016 by Martha Lindl.
Background Texture © by Iulia Shevchenko / Alamy Stock Photo.

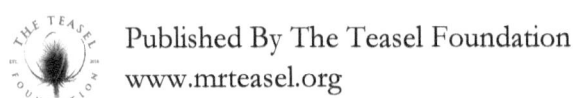 Published By The Teasel Foundation
www.mrteasel.org

The Teasel Foundation (a Public Benefit Corporation registered in the State of Montana, USA) is dedicated to the education of Lyme Disease

This Edition:
First Paperback Edition Published 2016.
ISBN: 978-0-692-73644-9 (Paperback).

Other Edition:
ISBN: 978-0-692-73643-2 (E-Book) (2016).

Other Language Editions:
ISBN : 978-0-692-78465-5 (E-Book) (French) (2016).
ISBN: 978-0-692-78466-2 (Paperback) (French) (2016).

Disclaimers

Medical Disclaimer

You understand that any information as found within this book is for general educational and informational purposes only. You understand that such information is not intended nor otherwise implied to be medical advice.

You understand that such information is by no means complete or exhaustive, and that as a result, such information does not encompass all conditions, disorders, health-related issues, or respective treatments. You understand that you should always consult your physician or other healthcare provider to determine the appropriateness of this information for your own situation or should you have any questions regarding a medical condition or treatment plan.

This information has not been evaluated or approved by the FDA and is not necessarily based on scientific evidence from any source. These statements have not been evaluated by the Food and Drug Administration (FDA). These products are intended to support general well-being and are not intended to treat, diagnose, mitigate, prevent, or cure any condition or disease.

You agree not to use any information in this book, including, but not limited to product descriptions, customer testimonials, etc. for the diagnosis and treatment of any health issue or for the prescription of any medication or treatment. You acknowledge that all customer testimonials as found on our Website are strictly the opinion of that person and any results such person may have achieved are solely individual in nature; your results may vary.

You understand that such information is based upon personal experience and is not a substitute for obtaining professional medical advice. You should always consult your physician or other healthcare provider before changing your diet or starting an exercise program.

In light of the foregoing, you understand and agree that we are not liable nor do we assume any liability for any information contained within this book as well as your reliance on it. In no event shall we be liable for direct, indirect, consequential, special, exemplary, or other damages related to your use of the information contained within this book.

Notice & Legal Disclaimer

For the purpose of this Notice & Legal Disclaimer the term "book" refers to all forms and editions of publication of *MR.TEASEL My Hero*, including but not limited to, e-book editions, digital & print editions, and abstracts or excerpts.

Trademarked names appear throughout this book. Rather than use a trademark symbol with every occurrence of a trademarked name, names are used in an editorial fashion, with no intention of infringement of the respective owner's trademark.

The information in this book is distributed on an "as is" basis, without warranty. Although every precaution has been taken in the preparation of this work, neither the author nor the publisher shall have any liability to any person or entity with respect to any loss or damage caused or alleged to be caused directly or indirectly by the information contained in this book.

For all matters related to this book, please contact the publisher, The Teasel Foundation, at www.mrteasel.org

Dedication

This Book Is Dedicated To The Tick Who Bit Me

Without that pivotal tick bite in the Summer of 2007, I never would have experienced this incredibly positive journey now unfolding in my life at age 64.

Ticks are part of nature, just as much as Wild Teasel. They both have their place on this planet. Yes, this one tiny tick brought profound personal destruction into my life, but without its bite, MR.TEASEL My Hero and none of this very important journey would have ever happened. I'm forever grateful for everything that's come into my life, both the good and the bad . . . because without the bad, sometimes the good never shows up . . . which I believe usually far outweighs the bad. That's one central truth expressed throughout this book. Yes, I do thank that tick. That tick brought about this book and changed my life forever.

Nature is supremely balanced. We humans are part of nature's balance . . . even if we sometimes forget that immutable fact. We must consciously allow the gifts of nature into our lives to be fully balanced human beings

Contents

Foreword   xvii

Dear Reader   xxi

Prologue   3

Introduction: The Possibilities   7
Everything's Possible,
From Ancient Cures To Stem Cell Therapy   8
Reality Time   11
More Back Story   13
Glucosamine & Chondroitin Sulfate   17
Adult Stem Cell Therapy – America   17
Stem Cell Therapy - European Union   20
Okay, Now My Head Is Really Getting Sore   2

Chapter 1: X-Rays Don't Lie!   27
Here We Shift Our Mental Gears, For A Moment   35
Let's Now Begin The Journey,
Knowing That We All Have Our Biases   37
My Grandma Told Me So   44
Authorship & Authority   49
A Little Bit Of Background On Me   50
How The Lyme Picture Came Into Focus   54

**Chapter 2: Pills, Potions, Lotions
& Other Sundry Concoctions In A Bottle**   59
Finding The Solution   66

Chapter 3: Pulp Fiction   69
The Rest Of The Story   72

Contents

And Then It All Ended 74
Time For A Change 75
A Jim Lindl Chest Thumping Editorial 75

Chapter 4: Weeds In The Ditch 81
The Cartilage & Lyme Killing Protocol Begins 85

Chapter 5: Heavy Artillery 89
I Can Feel This Stuff Working 92
A Flash Of Hope 100
It's In The Vibrations 103

Chapter 6: Teasel Lightning 111
Massive Fatigue, Fuzzy Brain, Low Motivation 113
I'm Getting Excited!!! 117
I'm Thankful 119

Chapter 7: The Waiting, The Healing 123

Chapter 8: My Green Mile 127
The Bellowing Bull 129
The First Heat Treatment 130
The Second Heat Treatment 133
The Detox Begins 134
Farting At Lake Helen 136

Chapter 9: Périgueux 143
The Teasel Ritual 145
Back To Earth For Another Day 146
The Surgeon's Meeting 147
Then It Got Worse 148

Contents

Then It Got Even Worse   150
Rewinding The Tapes   152

Chapter 10: It's Getting Dark Inside   161
Jim's New World Dictionary Definition Of Vulgarity   163
Back To My Brewing Stew   164
Laguna Beach Syndrome   166

Chapter 11; Full Moon Rising   175

Chapter 12: Reflection, Review, Reflection   179
The Last Six Months   181
Verbal Communication   187
The Sales Profession   187
My Communication Career Began Early   190
My First Sale   191
Two Wealthy Sisters   193
Early Lessons In Human Diplomacy   195
Towards A Grand Final Review   198
Oratory From The Pulpit   200
The Church   201
The Orator's Pause   203
The Final Review   207
The Grand Finale Of Changes In the Past 30 Days   212
Emotional Cleansing   217
My Big Surprise   219
Here's The Happy Beginning   229

Chapter 13: The Wild Horsetail Tea   231
Skin-Sack Of Bones   233
Muscular Balance Is Back   236

Contents

The Mother Of All Ganglions   239
The Bellowing Bull Returns   242
Frankincense Oil   243
A Change Of Heart   245
Time For More Communication
With The Main Power Plant   246

Chapter 14: Voices From The Wilderness   249
Knee Arthritis, Heal Thyself? New Research Says Yes!   253
Many Voices From The Wilderness   254

Chapter 15: Bowen Technique, Bowen Therapy   259
Traumatic Memory Can Be Locked Into Our Muscles   261
Back To The Back Spasm Problems   266
The Grand Finale With The Mullein   271

Chapter 16: Age 64   275
I Feel Young   281

Chapter 17: Stuck In Base Camp   287
Two Days With A Chain Saw On The River   289
Musings At The Water Mill In Dordogne   300
Where Is This Base Camp?   306
Why I'm Ready To Climb   311
Page 4/5 From MR.TEASEL My Hero   313
I'm Calling For New X-Rays   317

Chapter 18; Farewell Mr. Tease   319
Final Lyme Symptoms Update   321
A 100-Day Expedition To The Publishing Summit   322
My Waddington   323

Contents

The Route To The Top   323
The Teasel Foundation   324
Getting Started On Your Own Healing Journey   327
The Teasel Foundation's Founder, Jim Lindl,
Believes These Principles To Be Important & Noteworthy   332

Chapter 19: Working The 8-Point Plan   333
Back On The Teasel Elixir For Another 30 Days   336
A Ring Side Seat To The Teasel Foundation   337
Legal Work   337
Building A Website With Global Outreach   338
Teasel In America?   340
Delusion Vs Vision . . . There's A Difference   345
Start Simple & Grow   346
Frisbees Vs Glock 9's   347
Back To Building A Website   348
Cat's Claw & Sweet Wormwood Added For 30 Days   350
Business Summary   352
Teasel Bottleneck   353

Chapter 20: More X-Rays, More Blood Analysis   357
120 Kilos, 265 Pounds, 1.5 Kilometers, 4 Tons   360
The German Teasel Family   363
The Future Is Unfolding Right Here & Right Now   365
Concluding Remarks
On The Teasel Foundation Pre-Launch Activity   367
Summary Conclusion Of My Healing Journey   369

Epilogue   375
I'm Hopeful   377

Foreword

MR. TEASEL My Hero is authored by a long time patient of mine, Jim Lindl. It's a detailed account of his personal journey through the discovery and holistic treatment of his debilitating Lyme symptoms, as well as a raw, powerful and intriguing account of his life journey. *This book has changed my life*. In particular, it has changed the way I see my patients.

  I began private practice in 1980 and became a chiropractor because my very first treatment by a chiropractor, Dr. Al Dettloff, completely changed *my* life. At the age of 5 I took a bad fall, fractured my skull, and for the next 15 years had exertion asthma. I could not exercise without medication and experienced multiple trips to the ER in severe respiratory distress. Dr. Dettloff adjusted my atlas and in a flash, my respiratory issues vanished. You could say it was a miracle, but actually, it was science. Specifically, he executed relief from occipital/atlas mechanical traction against the respiratory centers on my lower brain stem and Cranial Nerve X (the Vagus Nerve). It's now 36 years later and I've treated well over 10,000 patients applying the same technology to qualified patients with previous injuries to their head and necks.

  I met Jim Lindl many years ago in California before he moved to retire in France. Last Fall, 2015, he called me from France to see me for treatment, thinking that his head and neck was out of alignment again, and assumed the resulting shift in his pelvic posture was the cause of his knee troubles.

When I saw the condition of Jim's knee, I knew it was more than mechanical pressure, and that there was definitely an infection in the joint! I referred Jim to Dr. David Halverstadt. The ability to diagnose the root of Jim's problem was right in his wheelhouse.

Honestly, I had no inclination whatsoever that Jim had Lyme disease. From the point of his Lyme diagnosis, Jim sought answers and solutions to somehow eradicate the disease from his life. And so began the daily journal which is now the highly detailed twenty-chapter e-book, *MR. TEASEL My Hero.*

Having followed the month by month healing journey of Jim since he left my office in September of 2015, and having watched the chapter by chapter story of *Mr. Teasel* unfold, my awareness meter has gone through the roof with patients that have been describing symptoms of Lyme disease. Since reading Jim's story, I have in just one month alone, directed twenty different patients to get tested for Lyme disease. Jim's fascinating story has had a profound effect on me and the way I consult with my patients.

Once this powerful and detailed book is published, I will suggest that each and every patient of mine visit the Teasel Foundation website and download *Mr. Teasel My Hero. If they have Lyme disease or Lyme disease symptoms, they could be in for the fight of their life. This book is a call to arms to fight back!* If they do not have Lyme disease, chances are, they know someone who does have Lyme but doesn't know that Lyme bacteria are infecting them. This book could bring them to that important awareness. We all love the story of how an individual struggles, and then prevails, against overwhelming odds. I am confident that anyone who reads this book will be motivated, moved and encouraged by Jim Lindl's victory over his debilitating Lyme disease symptoms.

If you are willing to completely commit to holistic natural self-healing and battle your Lyme disease, then you have a General to lead you: *Mr. Teasel.* Jim Lindl has laid out a simple step-by-step battle plan for you based on his personal, front line experience. This book is your boot camp. It requires only basic desire and firm determination to make it through. But, make it through you must if you are battling Lyme symptoms!

Dr. Jeff Blanchard, Precision Chiropractor Since 1980
Central Coast, California
May, 2016

Dear Reader

This is my first attempt writing any kind of book, and interesting to me being a non-fluent computer person, I've chosen the e-book format. Let me explain why.

There's a lot of material to cover in this book, almost overwhelming if a person tried to consume it all in a short period of time. I recognize there could possibly be a variety of personality types reading this somewhat lengthy story. People have different time constrains in their life, and in an effort to be helpful, I'd like to offer some thoughts about plowing all the way through to the very last sentence.

I'm neither a scientist, nor an expert on anything in particular, except old growth timber cutting, and certainly not qualified in any healing or medical fields where the reader should accept any of my conclusions. My writing here is just my story, and nothing more. My story in itself is about 102,276 words and 377 pages of simple story form writing that can be digested fairly easily chapter by chapter. That may be your best reading strategy if you have limited time and want to get the gist of this book's message. Just pass over the myriad of hyperlinks and suggested reading material that could bog you down and muddy the essence of my message.

However, if your interest is piqued along the way, and you want deeper clarification, expert thinking, state of the art medical updates, maybe a bit of entertainment, then by all means pause at those hyperlink junctures, click the blue cyber address and get the opinions and advice of fully qualified people most of which have PhD, DC, ND, MD, MS, Professor, or some government research agency logo tacked onto their name. These are people with decades of accumulated clinical and field experience, some of whose books I've read cover to cover multiple times, listened to their lectures, and traveled internationally between continents to gain their council.

They're offered in this book for verification, amplification, or clarification and hopefully simplification . . . to points I'm trying to highlight via my story. These are the people to listen to . . . not me. My story is here merely to provoke you into listening to some of these experts' messages. Think of me as an usher in a symphony hall directing you to the very best seats in the house to hear the music of the masters. That's my goal in this book.

My style is purposely breezy but yet deadly serious throughout. The entire book's undercurrent lays bare my dreaded respect for Lyme disease that's afflicted me for over seven years. When I began writing the book's introduction many weeks ago, my brain was struggling to get words off the keyboard up onto the screen. Fuzzy haphazard thinking and chronic stumbling body fatigue are hallmark symptoms of the Lyme bacterial spirochetes crossing the blood brain barrier and causing havoc in a person's deepest recesses of being.

As the pages unfold in the story and you move through the progression of time, you may detect a shift in my tone. I could feel it as I wrote from page to page and from day to day. Early in the first several chapters, particularly in the original draft before any editorial tempering, I could feel occasional latent vitriol and emotional cayenne oozing out of certain passages.

You may notice these tones in this final draft, but if not,

in the main they're still present, just lurking below the surface. If Lyme symptoms can cause a person to become a bit testy or even obnoxious and alienating, I do apologize, but I wanted the reader to feel my unvarnished mental temperament present at the time of writing. Those were my intentions while editing the original draft

Later in the writing, I could detect a shift away from nagging fears and hollowness within me, to more confidence, and belief as my health improved. At times later on in the narrative, I felt an almost *Hawkeye Pierce* tone of irreverent sassiness as I wrote. Some vulgarity creeps into the story by midpoint and it's not intentional or contrived. It just shows up. It remains as in the original because that expression is how I felt in the moment of writing.

Possibly, you'll detect some of these tonal changes as the book progresses. To me, it felt like my brain almost shape-shifted and gradually gained more clarity and focus as the Teasel Elixir and the healing protocol kicked in during the months-long writing and healing process. You'll be the judge of that opinion as the pages unfold.

I'm certain I've gone through some beneficial emotional cleansing as well as some significant physical changes, and an attitude shift during the writing, that I hope is interpreted not as cockiness, not as arrogance and not as I-told-you-so smugness, but . . . something different that I just can't quite identify. Maybe someday I'll understand all this shifting that's occurred during this period of my life. Maybe there's a spiritual component in this whirl of transformative process. Who knows for sure, but I hope you'll feel the changes on these pages as it gradually happened. I'm in the process of major healing during this writing, and I think it's evident beyond the mere written words

As I learned long ago, *Facts tell, Stories sell*. Dear Reader, my *story* is offered here in this book not to entertain you, not to enlighten you and not to educate you, but to *sell* you. I want to sell you a message of hope and healing that's waiting to be discovered.

Some of the links you'll find entertaining, some provocative, all I hope to be useful in supporting the theme in this book: Powerful holistic healing is hiding in plain sight for us all. We just need to keep our eyes peeled for the signals and messages along the journey . . . and allow these natural powers into our life.

MR. TEASEL
My Hero

Prologue

I've lived with Lyme disease symptoms for over seven years now, but it's not the imminent problem this writing deals with first. The opening focus is on my right knee. I can't walk. The knee joint is down to a grinding bone on bone contact you'll see shortly in an x-ray film taken two weeks ago. Lyme maladies, although most important, will be picked up later in the narrative. That's the sequence of how things are unfolding as I write.

Today is Saturday, November 21st, 2015 as I've begun to tap in these first few keystrokes. This may turn out to be a running daily event journal or maybe a full-blown book as time progresses. Time will tell. The actual day that this writing will be finished or released, I also don't know at this time. My future knee condition and the ongoing Lyme troubles will determine when, if ever it's published. It's impossible to predict. It depends on the healing mysteries of Naturopathy upon my debilitating cartilage and muscles infected by Lyme disease.

However, I guarantee this story will never leave this screen for the public to read if I have to go under the knife for my knee or my chronic fatigue continues unabated, or if the constant "lightning flashes" behind my eyes persist, and if the unusual blood pressure spikes and heart palpitations and other symptoms of malady continue like they have for many months.

Why would the persistence of these troubling signs stop me

from publishing this running journal of observations and notes? Well, because the working title above would be pure nonsense . . . and I don't plan on changing the subtitles or lying to the reader about what really happened. So in a very real sense, as I wrote this journal's working title today, and began this introductory passage, I'm optimistically predicting (hoping, dreaming) that a non-surgical knee repair and Lyme eradication will result from the healing direction I'm headed. I hope it works out for my sake as well as yours, and millions of other suffering people faced with arthritic induced knee surgery or the peculiar painful mysteries of Lyme disease.

A tall order to be sure, so why this optimism? Because I've researched and adopted a promising naturopathic alternative course other than surgery for my knee and a non-pharmacological treatment for the Lyme maladies that I believe will work. I'll begin this combined course of healing in about two weeks.

If everything goes as I expect, then this recorded personal journey will be released and, I hope, will help become a change-maker for future thinking about modern day self-healing. That's my goal in writing this journal: To make a difference.

Editor's note: The actual original working title was, *"How I Dodged A Bullet"*. *"Mr. Teasel My Hero"* was not born until page 109, after Jim's Lyme healing had progressed significantly.

Additionally, the confident passage below was added some time later than November 21st, after Jim's further Teasel research, his reading of Storl and introduction to stem cell treatment by the Colorado Clinic.

Dr. Storl had Lyme disease and brilliantly wrote about Lyme disease and its similarity to syphilis. He writes about Teasel (*dipsacus sylvestris*), self-healing and much more. He also beat his Lyme naturally. "So why not me too?" I thought. . . which is exactly what I plan on doing. You'll learn some interesting things about natural knee cartilage re-growth, Lyme disease, Teasel tinctures, self-healing, antibiotics, advanced nutrition, structural imbalances, the latest stem cell therapy, a brief passage about the French medical system and other sundry bits in this deeply personal journal about to unfold on your screen.

Let me explain further, what's going on and where this is all heading.

Introduction:
The Possibilities

I'm literally racing against the clock. In 26 short days, on December 16th at 9:00 a.m. in Périgueux, France I have an appointment with an orthopedic surgeon. I have a problem. A very big problem. The decisions I make in his office could be detrimental to the rest of my life. I need to think through this very clearly over the next few weeks. I'm acutely aware that major knee surgery is basically an amputation of two major boneheads that are replaced by implants that sometimes doesn't have a happy ending, especially with Lyme bacteria in the joint. I'll have to make a pivotal decision . . . in 26 days.

Edmonton, Alberta Canada, six days before Christmas, 1976, I went through L4-L5 back surgery at age 24. After that operation thirty-nine years ago, I wouldn't wish my never-ending back troubles on anybody. I know firsthand how post-surgery life can be compromised for a very long time. I really don't want to move my current knee disability into the permanent unfixable and miserable category. Not a good outcome but it's an inherent risk of major orthopedic surgery.

I'm a lifelong optimist by nature and have every confidence in the French Medical System and our Doctors here. This is where we live. This is our newly adopted retirement country of choice, and we're grateful we can live here. The Doctors here are as good as they get and, I believe, it's because France has a long history and cultural depth of good medicine and healing infused with their social compassion.

Call me old fashioned or naive, but I believe we reap what we sow. If that philosophy is true, then organizations like this one mentioned below, help explain the compassion in the French system. These folks are usually the first to arrive and the last to leave, long after all the TV cameras and politicians have rolled up and left the scene. This iconic international relief group, MSF, known in America as *Doctors Without Borders*, is a virtuous feedstock of crisis proven volunteer field Doctors circulated back into our French medical system. Doctors Without Borders (Wikipedia)

Everything's Possible, From Ancient Cures To Stem Cell Therapy

French heath care is both modern traditional and ancient holistic at the same time. After all, France *is* home to the Lourdes mystical healing waters made famous by the Catholic Church. Health spas and the tradition of mineral springs go back to the days of Roman Soldiers bathing their battle wounds in healing waters like the Vichy Celestine Source. If any of that spa pampering works, I say, go for it. About Vichy & Vichy-Célestins

And spas like the one linked below are just the beginning in Vichy. Vichy offers Opera & Spa weekends, Dinner, a Movie and Spa nights for two, and on and on . . . if you have the money. Vichy Célestins Spa Hotel

This town of 50,000 inhabitants was the occupational German Headquarters during WWII. "Good taste on their part," I say. Hence the name, "Vichy French Government" during World War II. Vichy was home to the indigenous French traitors and German Nazis who formed a provisional government for a few interesting war years. Some French avoid it today because of that conflicted dark history.

When driving through Vichy, we usually stop by their historic public fountain across from the park and tank up on free water like the rest of the locals. It tastes out of this world and I sleep with unbelievably vivid color dreams whenever I drink some of this direct out-of-the-ground natural unfiltered spring water that streams directly out of the hillside. The spring gushes out from a hillside of solid rock and is plumbed through a centuries-old ornate marble building where it flows to all the world for free. Any notion that the water is unsafe is quickly dispensed by sizing up the locals filling their jugs under a row of gorgeous bronze taps.

There must be something to it because wounded Roman soldiers weren't faking it, nor are the locals. I just haven't figured it out yet. But in the meantime, here is a provocative take on what the base mineral *Celestine* or Celestite, notably present in the Vichy Waters, can supposedly do for all of us. Maybe this is why I get so many dreams drinking the stuff. Who knows. Celestite (Celestine): The Stone That Can Help You Connect With Your Guardian Angel (Bliss Returned)

This is France and liberal thinking is *de rigueur* unless you live in parts of old France like we do. So I often stretch out and try to loosen up a little and emulate *Parisian French* myself and not automatically default to skepticism. I think it's healthy to once in a while speculate close to the fringe of one's current reality. That's how we explore interesting new territory and generate new ideas. It's probably why Christopher Columbus and his crew got to the Caribbean in 1492 when all the flat-earthers back home watched the sunset from their lounge chairs every day off the Spanish Coast and said, "That horizon, Dear Christopher, is the end of the line."

I say life can be sometimes more interesting if not life changing by keeping an open mind. The mind is like a parachute, it works beautifully, providing it's opened up before we hit the ground.

It's also readily apparent that France is seriously into old world herbal tinctures, and modern homeopathic formulas right beside mainstream physician prescribed big-time pharmacology brand names. Everywhere in France, it's not uncommon for a person picking wild mushrooms in the forest who has any questions about safety to take them to a pharmacy in their area. The local pharmacist will gladly look over a sack of their pickings and offer up copious amounts of good advice and expert opinions as to taste, texture and safety. I've done it several times myself. French people are definitely in tune with their health and beauty anyway possible . . . and it shows.

If a person gets sick, France is a great place to get help. Probably one of the best total health systems in the world. I've found that the French health care providers are very sincere and compassionate. Plus, everything, and I mean everything, is covered by our very affordable insurance: Testing, procedures, hospitals, clinics, meds, medical transportation, and rehab, all fully covered by insurance. No deductibles, no co-pays, one person to modern cheery hospital rooms, plus attentive nurses who have time to chat and talk nice. I should know.

I've personally been through an emergency high speed flashing blue light ambulance ride to our local hospital where I was studied, prodded, and poked for 14 agonizing hours in the ER. They didn't have to cut me open but the surgeon said he was ready to begin the next morning. Luckily, I dodged a gall bladder bullet that day and night, and then two years later, sailed through a hernia surgery here as well. So with that experience as background, I say the French medical system works very well. Good Doctors and good insurance are not an issue in this part of the world. I want my knees back functioning without trouble. "So knee surgery should be easy-peasy," I was thinking . . . up until about ten days ago.

That's when I discovered some new provocative holistic information in America that upended my built-in bias for surgery: Old thinking meets new thinking and creates a conflicting mental standoff. "What to do now?" I thought.

Reality Time

My right knee has been inflamed and swollen for about five months. Back in June, I bought my wife a badminton set for her birthday. I set it up for her all nice, proper, and inviting on our beautiful farm grounds all ready to go. That's as far as that idea ever went. I couldn't even chase that birdie a single step. At that moment, at age 63, I felt old; I felt broken and used up for the first time in my life . . . I couldn't even play badminton with my wife. A very simple retirement exercise and I couldn't begin to move. That reality began to tear at my inner strength and confidence as a human being. At that singular moment, I felt absolutely pathetic because never in my life before had I felt a tinge of sickliness or frailty and abject vulnerability like I did at that moment of truth. Quite the opposite. My entire life had been filled with robust physical activity of all types. I'm an on the go, physical person by nature and in that instant, my life changed. It was a terrible, sinking feeling that set in. I began to feel vulnerable for the second time in my life that sunny afternoon when I tried to chase that stinking birdie. I felt old for the first time in my life.

Now five and a half months later, I limp on a cane only limited distances, and usually with great difficulty and pain. I use a twin cylinder gas powered wheel chair to navigate our small farm. It's called a tractor riding mower. Our mailbox is 160 meters slightly uphill from the house and I don't fetch the morning mail anymore because of noticeable shortness of breath and significant knee pain. Sound sleep is impossible. By choice I don't take any pain killers at this time because I've read that pain is the most accurate early warning gauge as to when I'll need to go under the knife. Now I'm constantly thinking, "Not ready quite yet, I can take some more pain" . . . I've been here before at age 24, three months before back surgery in 1976.

I started writing this book because I firmly believe that last week I've actually found a nonsurgical holistic alternative program combined with an obscure herbal tincture, called "Teasel", that just may fix my worn out knee and the Lyme symptoms. I have no idea if this is going to work on me, but like one of the Doctors said, "Why not give it a shot." Surgery is forever once you have it done. No backing up. That's a very sobering thought at my age of 63 years. Good or bad I have to live with the outcome of major reconstructive surgery once I pull the trigger and say yes to the knife. I'm very clear on who is ultimately responsible here. Not the doctors, but me. Victim mentality isn't welcome into my brain at this stage of my life. It's never taken up residency yet in 63 years, but once it enters, I know it can be a damn hard tenant to chase back out even if it still pays the rent. I've seen it happen to a tough-as-nails logger who descended into victimhood and became a miserable soul because of his prisoner's mentality. He never shook it off. It killed his spirit along with his body. He was my trusted timber-cutting partner for a few years.

This book is about my journey. It'll document and link to a plethora of files, reports, books and sundry other obscurities of important information for anyone with knee troubles or Lyme bacteria swimming around in their body. Actually, anyone with joint troubles and not just those lined up for surgery in a few weeks. For just about everybody who runs, walks, climbs, stands, jumps, dances and jiggles and who has even a teeny tiny bit of joint clicking or occasional pain tweaks, this book is important. This includes tens of millions of Americans today, unfortunately many of them very young. That bit of joint clicking and tweaking pain is an early warning sign. I had those signs for many years.

My arthritic knee condition is what eventually happens to a lot of people, who either don't pay attention, or don't care, or simply don't know what's going on with those very important signals. Last count in the year 2010, 719,000 total knee replacements (TKR) were performed in the USA. In a few more years with the aging of the population and the continued decline of its overall national health condition, its forecast is that there'll be 3.5 million knee replacements per year in the USA. Those creaky sore joints of ours have devolved into a huge issue for far too many younger people today. And, most of its totally avoidable. We don't have to be limping around in pain. Little mystery why insurance rates are skyrocketing year after year for the past thirty years and people aren't happy with so many aspects of the American health care system today. Click here for some facts about Total Knee Replacement (TKR). Total Knee Replacement (Arthroplasty) (Beyond the Basics) (UpToDate.com)

Belatedly, I now know there are some excellent proven preventive things I could and should have done over the years. In this book there's going to be plenty of good information and numerous links to other resources on prevention as well as the crisis therapy I'm about to begin for my debilitating condition. Because of my previous executive leadership in a nutrition business I helped create, 23 years ago, I have a deep pipeline of experts and useful knowledge I can leverage and link into this book as back up resources for your consideration. Some of it's incredibly well proven but unfortunately not often known in the mainstream information flow. This book is going to be a robust compilation of expert health advice that you can tap into as well as a detailed journal of my nonsurgical holistic knee restoration and Lyme bacteria eradication.

All my life I've physically, mentally and spiritually explored and researched a lot of things and places and topics and "out there" concepts. It's just part of who I am, so it's not surprising that in the past several weeks I've unearthed some encouraging breakthroughs beyond my old thinking. These breakthroughs are the genesis of my optimism and new concrete plan for an alternative course of action. A nonsurgical holistic and naturopathic course of action.

More Back-Story

September last, I traveled specifically to California and consulted with two trusted Chiropractic Doctors I've known for years. That trip, although difficult and expensive, was very helpful. This wasn't a vacation. It cost us over seven thousand dollars and my wife had to roll me on a wheel chair through the airports and train stations getting from old France, through Paris, then San Francisco, and then by car to our final destination of San Luis Obispo California. Literally "Trains, Planes and Automobiles", both ways. Thirty-one hour straight haul, door to door. It was brutal but it was worth it because of what I learned about my knee.

I learned that I most probably had a Lyme bacterial infection going on in that bad knee for the past several years and still have it today. *Hello Jim Lindl !!!* I was both shocked and relieved because at least the whole picture was coming into better focus. I had a lot more going on than just a bum knee.

Then a month later after that California trip, another Internet-sourced Naturopathic Doctor gave me unusual confidence that, unlike what most doctors believe, the human body can grow sufficient new cartilage back to totally avoid surgery. In fact, he has done it for an uncountable number of patients! His forceful matter of fact belief in the possibility of full cartilage regeneration not using stem cell therapy was surprising news to me and pierced directly through my inherent skepticisms and biases. The resolved steady voice of his message resonated with me. As they say, "When the student is ready, the teacher shows up." Well I guess I was ready, because he sure was teaching me. I was beginning to evolve from a medical flat-earther to maybe thinking the healing waters bend over the horizon somehow.

I knew this Doctor was on to something and had to learn more. That's what this book is all about, but I don't know if he ever made all of his documented clinical results publicly available. He may not have, because of public ridicule or because he was simply too far outside any mainstream thinking at the time. Maybe it was because he would've attracted too much legal attention, but somebody did say his research and clinical results are all archived in the Smithsonian Institution in Washington, DC, where he's noted for his ground breaking medical understanding. Who knows the whole truth of the what, where and the why.

This Smithsonian feted Doctor was the genesis of this holistic journey and these writings. He was the spark that opened my mind. He cracked the door open and let some new light into my biased brain. He was the change maker in my thinking but he was only the beginning. It was one of his later day understudies, and an articulate Naturopathic Doctor in Minnesota, who introduced me to the idea of using teasel for Lyme disease.

After I was introduced to his video lecture on Lyme disease, there was no turning back. His name is Dr. Glidden N.D. You'll be formally introduced to him shortly, and together along with Dr. Storl, where his uncommon herbal wisdom, guidance and philosophy, will guide this thread of conviction and will help stitch together all these pages into a coherent usable map for the reader to follow into a world of better health and healing. Most Medical Doctors I've read don't think that it's possible to re-grow sufficient new cartilage fast enough to overcome the constant grinding down of the old cartilage in our joints. Can't be done. Not with pills, potions, lotions, transplant bone plugs, or drilled helper growth holes. Period, *unless* it's adult stem cell transplant therapy. "When the patent has Lyme disease, they're all probably right," I thought. Some people say Lyme has no bearing on knee cartilage degeneration, that it doesn't matter. I'm pretty sure in my case it has. "This is all getting very confusing and conflicting," I thought.

For sure, there are a bunch of other exotic procedures available in some expensive and interesting clinics around the world that'll be glad to use you as a guinea pig if you have enough money. Sorry, that's not for me. Besides, I'm not rich. I need something simple that I can do now. Something that works. Next subject please. The clock is ticking... December 16th, is fast approaching and that orthopedic surgeon is waiting to have a talk with my knee.

Glucosamine & Chondroitin Sulfate

Here is an extensive National Institute of Health double-blind medical study that proved treatment with the widely touted combination of Glucosamine and Chondroitin sulfate supplementation for knee/joint disorders is ineffective. I'm not so sure, but their study seems to indicate it just doesn't work. I know there are plenty of vitamin hawkers who swear by the stuff. Even Stem cell MDs and their clinics suggest it, and peddle it post procedure before you go out the door with a new stem cell knee job. One-stop shopping, I guess. Who knows. Sometimes I think they're just *"practicing medicine"* on us all. Q&A's - Glucosamine/Chondroitin Arthritis Intervention Trial Primary Study, May 2002 (NCCIH)

This study was conducted on people all over the age of 40 with an average age of 59. The placebo subgroup was no better or worse off taking sugar pills. So this holistic food Supplement route doesn't seem promising on the surface based on this particular report, which goes against the grain of a lot of Glu/Chon Sulfate believers.

Adult Stem Cell Therapy - America

Maybe adult stem cell therapy in the future is the answer. It's exciting but sketchy according to some MDs in America who want more long term testing to be sure that it's safe. Although this clinical therapy seems to be gaining traction pretty quickly, I need something I can believe in today. Something that I can trust and afford. The CDC isn't holding the door wide open to willy-nilly, run and gun stem cell treatment, but you can go offshore for stem cell exotica, if that's your cup of tea. Linked below is a very interesting news article from over five years ago about the early success by some pioneers in stem cell treatment out of Denver. Please read it. There are some excellent further links embedded in this article that can expand our understanding the benefits and how it works. This is a good start to understanding the origins and direction of stem cell therapy for joint repair. I'm signed up for this particular clinic's webinar November 30, 2015. It sounds interesting and informative and I'll report more on it after the broadcast. I've already posted some pre lecture questions for their Doctors. Stem-Cell Therapy Feels Food & Drug Administration's Pinch, The Denver Post, April 12, 2010

Five years later, linked below is the current commercial evolution and growth of that same original Doctor's stem cell clinic in Denver and the future direction it's being guided. As of late November, 2015, this clinical group alone is up to 22,000 plus stem cell treatments, mostly knee-jobs since 2005. Very worthwhile for all of us to follow Doctors and clinical developments like these folks who are pioneering for all of us. It may be in our future to eventually eliminate most orthopedic joint surgeries. They seem to think so and it does look promising even if it costs a small down payment on a new home and isn't covered by insurance because it's not an *approved* procedure.

Approved by whom I don't know, but apparently not by the insurance gods on high who divvy up our expensive monthly premiums. A reluctant official full-blown medical establishment endorsement of stem cell treatments simply means one thing to me: Money. Too much money is sloshing among certain people to rock the boat. To me, reluctant insurance approval just means folks like this Denver Clinic are nicely hijacking somebody else's lucrative orthopedic surgery lunch money through medical turf encroachment, and the politics of overpriced medicine is holding the door shut on stem cell medicine for as long as possible . . . in my opinion. Nothing new under the sun . . . Old medical money likes the cushy ride they fought hard for in DC. I don't blame them. It's just good business if not good medicine.

There's a rational transformation coming for effective American healthcare delivery, but probably not in my lifetime. I expect that because of eventual medical economic burnout the changes will be forced upon us and that might begin with means testing for Medicare. I can see it coming for many in my generation. Us schmucks who tucked away a small purse for a rainy day will wonder how come were getting wet under the government's social protective big top. I'm prepared for the transition. We're not covered by American Medicare now in France and we'll just have to pay our own freight like the productive class always has in the past . . . With our own hard work up to the finish line.

Here are the Denver people who have done over 22,000 (as of November, 2015) stem cell jobs on knees, hips, backs, etc. Stem Cell Therapies For Arthritis & Joint Injuries (Regenexx)

My Concerns With Stem Cell Treatment Are Several:

1) One treatment may work and last for some time but if, I have a structural alignment condition or internal health condition like Lyme bacteria that caused my knee joint to

degenerate in the first place, what is to prevent failure from recurring? In other words, this stem cell cartilage re-growth may work, but my body may just as rapidly grind it all off again and I'll be back at the same painful place that I'm now. That's the reason why knee replacements only last ten to fifteen years. They wear out. I want to make sure I'm getting to the root cause of my knee failure as well as get a repair job... Not a quick temporary fix but a total long-term healthy solution.

2) The cost can be substantial and isn't covered by insurance.

3) Even though I have to pay up front, there's no guarantee that the stem cells will regenerate fast enough in my body to rebuild. Everybody's body is different. This procedure isn't like implanting some titanium mechanical devise.

4) These clinics are quick to trot out their patient successes with inspiring video testimonies, but I wonder what their success ratio is across the totality of all treated patients? I'm not clear about that statistic yet. I'll ask it on the webinar Monday.

Stem Cell Therapy - European Union

I like the following site for its treasure trove of education about stem cell development in Europe. If you're in North America reading this book, this site will give you a feel for the differences and the similarities of medical treatment philosophies, state of research, and direction of application in Europe vs. The United States.

This is a very robust resource for anybody anywhere in the world considering this important future of medicine. It's in six languages, English included, so everybody is covered.

Euro Stem Cell (Europe's Stem Cell Hub)

And finally, the *coup de grace*, to cool your jets about running out and getting the latest quick fix at your local stem cell shop around the corner with a limited track record.

This link is from a UC Davis Medical school professor interview. (Spoiler Alert!) He admits he's biased and skeptical. Don't watch this one if you're all gung-ho to seed your joints with some stem cells. You might back out. From the Huffington Post Interview in California: *Considering A Stem Cell Treatment From A Clinic? . . . HuffPost Healthy Living, September 24, 2012*

To be fair to everybody, this interview was three years ago and that's almost like the dark ages in the fast-moving field of Biomedical Science. He talks about his blog site. If he still has one that may be a forum to get his current thinking. He was an assistant professor and medical researcher of note as of 2012.

But I always ask myself about anybody I read on either side of the fence, "Do people, like this professor, get funding by somebody to do outside work?" If so, by whom? Who is the benefactor or patron saint of some "scientific" study? Believe me I'm not suggesting this particular person or anybody else is on the gravy train of funded research. But to not ask and know the authors' roots of financial sustenance and core philosophies, portends the distinct possibly of bamboozlement. Look at the DC beltway empire builders, the ultimate charade of self-interest bamboozlement taken to a high spiritual level. Dear Reader, there's a plague out there of self-interested bias in the medical world as well as other places. There's too much gravy money involved to think otherwise. I expect you to ask no less about me as you read these pages . . . Who benefits?

This link below is an eye-opening article on doctor/medical establishment payola written by a well-known doctor himself! Embedded in this article is another link to a new government watchdog where you can enter any doctor's name in America and find out if they're being paid by drug or devices companies to push their particular products. Very revealing how much money is sloshing around the system. Some of the Physician payoffs are staggering. This article *confirms my bias* of one reason why the American system of medicine is so overpriced relative to the rest of the world: Payola, which is the title of this documented article. Payola In Medicine - Insights Into The Murky Side Of Patient Care (Regenexx)

Recently I met a man with a fully completed hip surgery performed in Limoges, France, paid for with cash. He's a retired British gentleman who lived and worked in Dubai for the past 45 years. He's 78 years old, now lives in our community, and just got the operation done. Because he has neither British National Health coverage, nor French Universal Health coverage, he operates bare-naked with no insurance and pays cash as he goes. The total cost for that hip, everything included . . . 7,500 Euros, about $8,300. I have the name of his orthopedic surgeon and clinic who also offered him a stem cell hip repair option in lieu of surgery, which he declined, because he didn't understand how stem cells work. Mechanical titanium parts sounded efficient and logical to him.

This newly rebuilt patient drove himself up to our local Irish pub *ten days* after surgery for his first beer. I found all this out because I drank one with him that night. "Who benefits?" I wondered, from a $60,000 hip surgery in some hospitals of the world, Dear Reader? Who benefits? One modern country charges 8,000 dollars and another country is 60,000 dollars both with equivalent professional excellence and with long-standing track records. Why the big difference? I try to measure carefully the voracity and biases of printed and spoken thought and expect you'll do no less as you turn these pages.

Okay, Now My Head Is Really Getting Sore!

"So, who does a person listen to?" I thought. I'm not so sure any of these healers, whoever they are, have all the optimal or complete answers. There are some very serious differences of opinions out there that can whipsaw a person's reasoning. I don't want to get sucked into an emotional solution that's sub-optimal for me and might regret later.

Nonetheless, all this back and forth has stimulated my belief and confidence that there's strong merit to go ahead with my alternative naturopathic plan that'll eliminate the need for a surgical procedure on my knee and strengthen all my joints simultaneously and not just the badly deteriorated right knee. It's a holistic approach, non-invasive and relatively inexpensive. I expect to see initial results within 60 to 90 days. That's my expectation. You'll read all about my progress in real time as it unfolds over the next few months.

Through all this I've learned there's compelling research, information and clinical confirmation that there are some complex holistic functions that the human body can latch onto and rebuild the knee joint and kick out nasty Lyme disease all at the same time.

This e-book will provide you with extensive information, links and running progress reports as I climb this mountain in front of your attentive reading glasses. You're going to witness each and every twist, turn, and stumble I take along the way. That's the objective of this book. To document a crystal clear guided map of the path I'm now taking so others can follow it themselves if it makes logical, truthful, healthy sense to the reader.

I've decided to construct these pages with different types of readers in mind. For the time-challenged individual who wants just an abbreviated version and wants to get right to essential curative points in a couple of hours, they can skip the hyperlinks and other suggested supplemental reading for now. After an initial cruise through the pages, they can then back track to all the hyperlinks to study, ponder, and learn much more. For the serious student who wants to fully wade and wallow in the many subplots to the main story, it could take a couple of months to navigate this swamp of writing. You'll be able to access important books and study the doctors, herbalists, scientists, clinics and sundry soothsayers I'm going to trot out for consideration. I look at all these resources as silent teachers patiently waiting to enlighten us all. They're our guides and cheerleaders. If you too choose to climb your own challenging health mountain someday, these same guides are waiting to help you too. That's why they're included in this book. There's some powerful and wise teaching available in the links and references sprinkled throughout the book. So . . . I suspect this book will be pretty extensive when completed. I want it to be detailed, accurate, not entertaining, but full of valuable interesting information every step of the way in a breezy crosscut style with occasional light decoration to keep the reader engaged for the important punch lines that I know can possibly change lives for the better.

Hopefully my writing style doesn't turn off the readers'

interest before they get to those important nuggets embedded in these pages. It would be a tragedy for me as a writer and a fellow human being to have found solutions to better myself, but left the reader out in the cold because of my verbosity. Hopefully you put up with me so you can follow along, avoid surgery, kill off your Lyme disease once and for all or better yet, learn some preventive steps to never get into the painful situation I'm in now and live a healthy and happy pain-free mobile life.

If you want to dispatch with my pulp verbiage and are a bottom line centric information digester who needs to cut to the quick for those magic bullet solutions for Lyme troubles or suspected Lyme troubles, you need to seek the star of this book immediately, Mr. Teasel. He is presented to all the world in his full glory in Chapter 4, which begins on Page 61. That'll take you to the front of the class, probably unprepared, but maybe where you need to be, if you want to chew through my breezy pages *à la carte*. If I had precious little time to waste, I'd skip everything in this book except two things:

Anything to do with teasel tinctures and Dr. Wolf-Dieter Storl. Storl is a world renowned Teasel Expert. He, teasel tincture, and a few other important items, have your back if you have Lyme disease.

Chapter 1:
X-Rays Don't Lie!

As I sit at my desk and write, it's now Tuesday, November 24th, 2015. 22 days to my December 16th morning appointment with the surgeon in Périgueux.

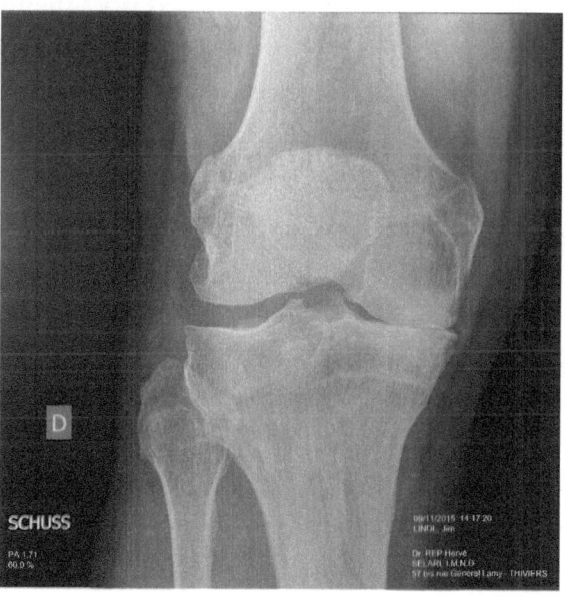

My Right Knee X-Ray, November 09, 2015
© 2016 Jim Lindl

Any radiologist in the world could take one look at this knee joint and see the problem. I learned later, on December 16, from an Orthopedic Surgeon, this is a Stage 4 Condition, ready for replacement.

I certainly know there's a problem even without these pictures because I can't walk! The knee pain is killing me. This is the bone on bone physical reality.

This current x-ray is my beginning point of holistic therapy to attempt rebuilding that joint back to full mobility. I expect to start the journey by December 10th, at the latest. Hopefully sooner because my pain clock is ticking louder each day and the idea of the knife is a disturbing thought.

Take a look at the text details on the films. My name, the date, the doctor's name, the radiologist in our local town. Pretty easy facts to verify. Like I said in the introduction, everything will be accurate, detailed and documented in this book. This x-ray of my right knee tells it all. It's bone on bone degeneration. It hurts like hell because there's no cartilage left in critical places where it's needed.

There's also a detailed written analysis of this x-ray by the radiologist that will be made available for any Doctor who may want to read and study these observations and notes. It's all in French, so you'll need a good French medical translator. I can help you locate one if you're a doctor and want to review their analysis. You can contact me at: jimlindl@mrteasel.org

For everybody else, even if it was in English, it's all technical bone/knee/ joint technical Doctor Talk. I haven't a clue what it all means. My everyday family doctor here just said to me, "You have a problem and that cartilage will never grow back." I already suspected that myself, and knew why he was so adamant. The medical research studies he reads say it just can't be done. I read some similar studies like the one linked earlier. They say it just can't be done effectively with our current medical knowledge.

I was bitten just above the knee joint on the RHS by a tick in September, 2007, about 12 months before this next x-ray

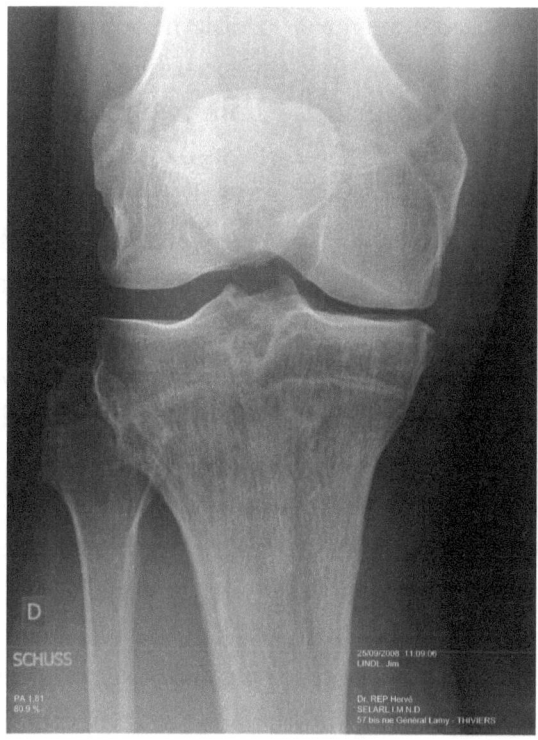

My Right Knee X-Ray, September 25, 2008
© 2016 Jim Lindl

Spot the difference? This second x-ray is from the same clinic, same radiologist, but taken almost exactly 7 years earlier. From these earlier x-rays it's evident there was some deterioration taking place.

Days after this x-ray I got blood work results that indicated no problem with Lyme bacteria, and otherwise in 100% perfect health.

Meanwhile my mobility and joint pain began to seriously amplify about the time frame of this x-ray, September, 2008, twelve months after the tick bite.

I learned later, on December 16th, 2015, that this joint, in September 2008, had 90% cartilage remaining and only about 10% cartilage degeneration, 1 year after the tick bite.

My knees were never a problem before in my entire lifetime until after that tick bite in France, Fall of 2007. I started using a walking stick within two months of the bite, and about a year after the bite, it was bad enough to see a local doctor. The pain was constant, so this doctor in September, 2008, called for x-rays that you see here. I've used a beautiful birch walking stick most days ever since. It has become part of my old man identify.

At the time of that first x-ray, September, 2008, I was prescribed a set of crutches and prescription meds because that right knee was extremely painful. I tried the pharmacology route for a while but then later found out about all the serious side effects after my own blood pressure shot up: Side effects like blood clots, heart attacks, strokes and a bunch of other wicked stuff was common. I believe they've limited the use of that specific med in most countries by now. Lawsuits tend to do that and the doctors here don't talk about using it anymore. The pain went away by Spring of 2009, only for it to periodically return with a vengeance.

I eventually buried those crutches in the town dump and went back to the birch stick. Old French men use sticks, not crutches. I became a happy stick man. Finally, in Spring of 2015 the internal heat like pain gripped my knee permanently. That's when my walking ability deteriorated significantly. It's also the time frame when the lightning flashes in the eyes, the shortness of breath, the heart palpitations, and significant general overall muscle weakness entered the picture permanently. That was all in early Spring, 2015.

I remember very clearly the defining moment I knew I was in serious trouble. We were in the 16th arrondissement of Paris, in mid-April, 2015. Parking is almost impossible in Paris especially in that area, but thanks to our dog who was with us, we had to find a quiet shady location for him, to leave him alone in the car for a few hours. Shady Paris parking is virtually impossible to find anywhere but serendipity struck again . . . a common theme in my life. Things that I need tend to always show up at the right time . . . if I pay attention. We found some trophy dog parking right across from the horse track.

It was on this Paris trip that I realized for the first time I had a very serious issue with my knee and my health state generally. We parked, set out walking toward Starbucks, less than a mile, and I couldn't make it. Stick or no stick. I had walked to failure, which reminded me of my ambitious mountaineering days: We would climb very hard technical alpine routes and push ourselves until we approached our mental or physical failure limits. I found mine in Paris that day walking to Starbucks.

I sat down on a park bench; while my wife went on to fetch us the goodies. She returned. That was the last time I ever walked in Paris. Before that trip, it wasn't unusual for us to walk the streets of Paris for hours upon hours, miles upon miles and I knew I was in trouble that day. I couldn't walk 500 yards down a dead level sidewalk to get a cup of coffee. My wife drove us out of Paris that day. I became the passenger.

I write very consciously about that tick bite now . . . however . . . I never made the correlation between the tick bite and my knee pain until September 15, 2015 after consulting with a trusted California Doctor. In fact, I forgot all about ever being bitten by a tick until this California Doctor did an extremely thorough patient interview over two separate hour-long appointments.

Four years before the 2008 knee x-ray I had climbed

Yosemite's Half Dome, from Camp Curry to summit and back to Camp Curry in one sustained 14-hour push without any thought of cartilage trouble brewing. Half Dome is a serious sustained rock route by any definition and in our down climb on the way out we encountered some serious early winter heavy weather that enveloped the valley.

Three years later, I had a tick bite on that knee in the x-ray. One year after the bite, I was walking with a cane and on pain medication. Today I'm facing surgery because I can barely make it to the garage and back carrying some firewood in my arms. Something drastic was happening in that knee joint to cause all this deterioration and I don't believe it came from being a peaceful simple gardener in France these past seven years. That knee joint lasted a lifetime of punishment and then suddenly fell apart with bone-to-bone contact in 7 years of light gardening? I don't think that's logical.

I never in my lifetime had trouble before with my knees . . . so, was it the tick bite? . . . or something else. Something has happened to my overall muscle system that's sucking the life out of me. My wife can lift groceries out of the car easily but I hesitate with one 20-pound bag. I'm short of breath, have eye flashes and heart palpitations and the doctors tell me they can find nothing wrong with me. This is the hardest mountain of my life I'm climbing right now as I sit at this computer. It's like my energy, my spirit, and my soul had been devoured by unknown forces.

My Half Dome climbing partner and friend died in a fast freight train wreck in Northern Idaho, August 25 this past summer. It was an unprotected level crossing. He got T-boned on the driver's side. He never saw it coming. Instant death . . . thankfully he never suffered. I miss him. He was a special friend. We talked on the phone in April about my failing health and about his new bright happy life in Northern Idaho. He was never happier in his life. A peaceful soul he was. He never so much as stubbed his big toe up high in the mountains.

This is the last mountain I shared with my friend. We left the park in the dark that night and parted our ways for the last time before I moved on to France. He smiles on us all today. I'm grateful for all the special mountain magic we experienced together up high. Hiking Half Dome Video (from National Park Service) and A Renewal Of Life On The Edge Of Death, NY Times, April 24, 2005

I'm done using ibuprofen after reading this article: American Heart Association Warns Of The Risks of NSAID Use (Regenexx)

So this is my current situation. Right now, I'm scheduled to see the orthopedic surgeon in 25 days. I know where that road leads me and I have major concerns about going under surgery with potential Lyme bacteria in the joint complicating post-operative recovery. Like another doctor told me long ago, once you go under the knife, there's no backing up.

Because of my growing concerns, I've seriously engaged in massive action seeking a realistic alternative. But where and what?

Well I've found it and I've now been developing my alternative plan. That's what this book will document and plug you into . . . my plan of action.

I expect to include the final x-rays, doctors' comments with their analysis and my own thoughts at the end of the book. I hope we're all looking at a remarkable transformation and celebration of confirming films. Even if you may think I'm stretching the truth as you follow this detailed narrative in the ensuing Chapter 1: X-Rays Don't Lie

That badminton birdie doesn't lie either. I also expect to include a video clip of me chasing that birdie before the end of this story

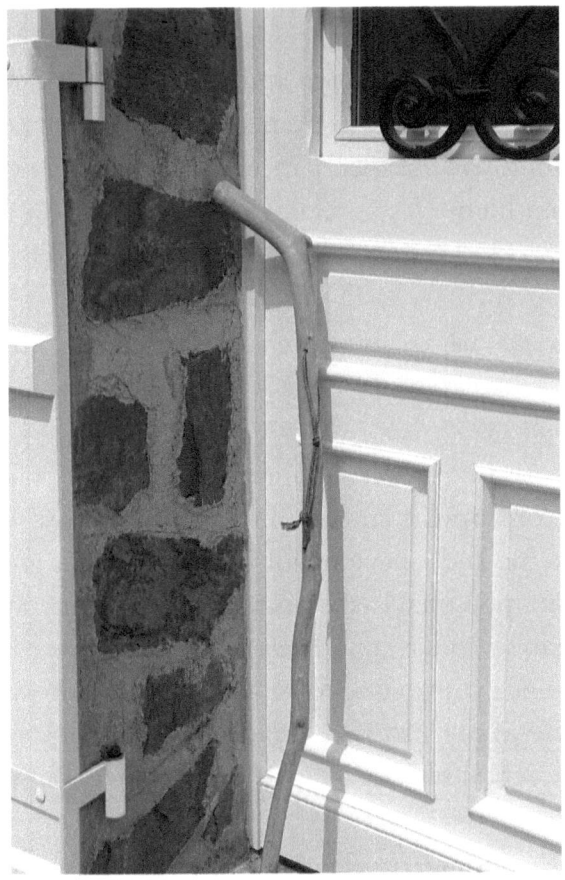

My Faithful Birch Walking Stick

Here We Shift Our Mental Gears, For A Moment

This segment is a heads-up mental preparation before diving into the ensuing chapters. Let's begin.

If I was to use the colloquial expressions, Head in the Sand, Block Head, Biased, Thinking inside a Square Box, Prejudiced, Narrow Minded, Intolerant Thinker, and Know-it-all, what comes to mind? Those aren't very becoming expressions that I just used. But unfortunately, sometimes we as human beings are programmed with the tendency to stick to ideas and philosophies we hold dear but may not be completely serving us. This type of thinking process is all very human. The fancy psychological term is Confirmation Bias (CB).

What is Confirmation Bias? Here's one of the best explanations I've read. Beware before you click on unless you have a bit of coffee time to sip and ponder. Confirmation Bias (Wikipedia)

You're maybe asking yourself, "Why is he going into this other stuff? I thought he was going to talk about knee surgery alternatives and beating the crap out of his Lyme bacteria?" Believe me, this is important. Although I've got time on my hands waiting until December 16th, these words aren't just page pulp written for decoration or entertainment.

In fact, this short narrative section may be *the* master key for you gaining your own personal health objectives out of this book. If you can truly hold in check any lurking long held biases while reading this book, you'll likely have some major breakthroughs as you delve deeper into all the linked resources. In fact, I guarantee it. There are some pretty interesting things in this book that I'm positive, you're unaware that might press against the grain of your own biases.

This book will be exposing and exploring some ideas and some thinking that may be quite provocative or even destructive to your current philosophies. We as human beings all have a tendency to keep thinking along the same old lines that have shaped and served our lives. And the more different, difficult, unconventional or even radical that some information is (no matter how useful); we usually don't want to read it, hear it or think about it. In fact if we have a well-developed point of view, we tend to read-only authors, seek other knowledge sources or associate with people who are like-minded to support that viewpoint even further. That's what *confirmation bias* is all about. I have it, and everybody usually has it to some degree.

Ask a Democrat what time a day it is, and then ask a Republican what's the time and you get two different answers, because they can't agree on using the same clock. That's what a very legitimate and rational-based bias looks like. They argue over the clock but not the definition of time, unless of course, they went to Oxford and their name is Bill. Then any type of irrational argument works and it all goes downhill from there into irrational biases to pure delusional obfuscation and bamboozlement.

Unfortunately, our self-imposed CB can be a costly mental trap. It thwarts us from discovering and exploring wonderful positive alternatives in life. That's what thinking outside the box is all about. But truly independent self-directed thinking is difficult and slows down at a very early age. We're all socially programmed to conform very early in life. It's usually easier to get along if we go along by marching to the popular drummers that surround our life and our thinking.

For me, I've had a major 23 year well developed "head in the sand" CB that jammed up my thinking until just last week. You'll read about it by the end of this chapter. If I had stayed stuck in my old paradigm, this book would never have had the *possibility* of a happy ending. Instead, I'd be heading to the operating room very soon and my knee would've been carved up like a Christmas Goose. It's now November 28, 2015 when I write this. The clock is ticking . . . That appointment is now only 17 days away and I can't yet begin my holistic program.

It's very hard to break out of our molded thinking unless we are forced. I was forced to open my mind up by this impending knee surgery. We are people of patterns and repetition who like to follow formulas and Gurus whether by habit, convenience, social convention, family stigma, or workplace requirements and financial constraints. Some earnest hopeful change-makers suggest our thinking is nefariously directed by mass media propaganda and Big Brother dominance. Other learned academics think of us humans as nothing more than unenlightened sheep. Whatever the myriad of reasons . . . I call it life. The bottom line is that we all have to deal with our patterned thinking in order to find alternatives that can serve us better.

Let's Now Begin the Journey, Knowing That We All Have Our Biases

Peter Egoscue: I'd be extremely surprised if you've ever run across that name before. Why? Well for starters you most likely wouldn't have sore clicking joints or even worse, be facing surgery like the one I'm facing right now if you had been introduced to him.

Jack Nicklaus? You've probably heard of him. For our younger non-golfing readers here's an inspiring link to his Bio. Jack Nicklaus Bio (Wikipedia)

Tiger may be a stellar golfer, but Jack is much more to me than just one of the best golfers of all time. He's an inspiration.

What if I suggested that you read a book Pete wrote about joint pain, joint surgeries, steroid treatments, chiropractors, athletic performance, athletic malfunction and some other really scary stuff about the current epidemic state of joint malfunction in America? Would you click onto Amazon right now to buy it and read it? Probably not. There are hundreds of books like his out there. A new obnoxious Guru seems to show up on late night infomercials all too often as a constant reminder for us to just steer clear of it all.

I wish I had read Pete's book before it was too late for my knees. In fact, one of Pete's earliest books was gifted to me long before I ran into my big knee troubles. It was a book quietly recommended by a trusted Doctor, who has become more like a family friend over the years. Why didn't I read it? Probably because of certain thick headed thinking on my part. Maybe at the time this compassionate benefactor needed to be more forceful and impress the need to study Pete's core messages in the book. Unfortunately, for me that's not this Doctors style. He's a kind and gentle soul who likes to help and heal. I wish now he would've banged me on the head and severely lectured about the Egoscue Method when he kindly handed me the book ten years ago . . . just like he has to hundreds of others. Unfortunately, I only glanced through this book and never took it to heart. It collected dust until this past June.

Jack Nicklaus, the famous golfer, opens Pete's first book

with a glowing forward. Why?

According to Jack, Pete changed his whole life. Jack was pretty well done golfing because of his debilitating back troubles. He wanted to stay in the game at the professional level but he was washed up with pain and maladies beyond any Doctors ability at the time. Jack followed Pete's advice . . . A unique stretching routine and nothing else. No drugs, no vitamins, no Chiropractors, no surgery, no nothing and it cost Jack nothing but a little bit of his time over a few months. It changed his life. He tells you his story in that introduction.

Here's a little bit about Pete himself. He's a Vietnam Vet, Marine Combat Officer, shot up pretty bad, went through hell and back with all the rehab, and was still a mess after being discharged from all the hospitals.

After going into his own intense research to understand the source of his chronic pain, he developed a unique method to clean pain out of his system, and then prevent it from ever coming back. Pete eventually cured himself when no one else had a solution. Ditto for tens of thousands of Pete's followers since them. He opened a clinic in San Diego where the lame and the infirm started coming in by the droves, including Jack Nicklaus, along with a ton of other celebrity athletes who had tried everything money could buy to get healed. Most people seemed to find Pete like me, pretty late in their joint troubles and then probably wished they had found him years sooner. Later on Pete wrote a couple of books and did a radio show for years before he slowed down, but yet, you probably never heard of him because he was never personally recommended to you. Just like you've probably never heard the names Glidden, or Storl or Regenexx or Lindl or Teasel. You likely found you way to this e-book because somebody suggested you take a look.

That's how CB works. We can stay tuned out and turned off to valuable information that surrounds us constantly, unless somebody hits us over the head to pay attention. Confirmation Bias is a tough nut to crack because we like to keep dancing to the familiar drummers we know and trust. I like to say, "Often times, important and beneficial information is so close to our nose, it's totally out of focus, and we can't begin to see it."

What is Pete's magic method all about? Stretching. Yep, stretching, but it's a unique gentle systematic routine that virtually anybody can do almost anywhere, all for free. Buy his first two books for less than twenty bucks and all the rest is free. No clinical visits, no pills, potions, lotions, sweat lodges or voodoo modalities that may scare you back to a church confessional. Simple, technical stretching routines very well illustrated that he developed as a crippled Vietnam Vet. About 15 different ones in total. That's what allowed Jack Nicklaus to get back onto the golf course without back surgery. It's all in the book. If you're a golfer, you'll find out why it can cure your hook or slice because the answer usually is in your posture and not a more expensive coach or different golf clubs. The magic secret is all in our general posture and correct joint alignment. Did you observe how your thinking subtly shifted while reading this passage?

I'm sure if I tried to *sell* you this passage without mentioning a famous celebrity golfer who endorsed Pete, you may have taken a pass on reading Pete Egoscue's book. Now you may take a look. That's how CB works. Our thinking is often positively nudged by strong testimonies and truthful endorsements that are directly linked to our personal needs. This book I'm writing is designed to use my anticipated successful knee outcome as a proof positive example to nudge the reader to look at holistic alternatives outlined in this book.

In his second updated edition published six years later in 1998, Pete is endorsed by Anthony Robins of some contemporary fame, Theodor Forstmann the New York Billionaire deal-maker extraordinaire along with the noted spiritualist and healer, Dr. Deepak Chopra among other luminaries who came through his door for treatment.

If it were me, I'd buy both of his books because they're somewhat different. I still like the original better for its complete total body routines. By the time he wrote the second edition, I suspect that Pete may have found the average person wasn't able or willing to invest the full hour plus it takes do a complete Condition II or Condition III session. In the second book he breaks out these full routines into what I call "stretching-light" for the time challenged. I'm sure they're just as effective but I like the total body approach better. Only Pete could tell you the reasons for modifying the routines.

My first recommendation for your own health maintenance and for absolutely everybody out there whether they're fully fit or broken and limping like me, fat or skinny, athlete or couch potato, young or old, is to purchase these two books by Pete Egoscue. Read them and you'll be educated why most of us are walking time bombs heading into the operating room just like me. Last count 43 million American have arthritic joint deterioration and are in pain. It's an epidemic.

I'm a classic case of a lifetime all-around-fit, healthy and a multi-activity person, who eats a very clean diet, pays attention to their health, has never been overweight, and has tried to live conservatively. Nonetheless, the scalpel and those pretty nurses are calling me in Périgueux. Something went wrong with my program and Pete goes a long way toward enlightening us all what is happening with our joints.

You may be asking me if I do these routine stretches now with a hopelessly bad right knee. Of course I do! "Why?" you may ask. Very simple: I still have two ankles, one good knee, two hip sockets, a damaged spinal column, two elbows and two shoulders and a neck and skull that I want to keep out of the hospital.

I wish I had read Pete's book years ago before I got into this mess. Although the book was gifted to me by a trusted Chiropractor I've known for years, I never read it until it was too late. I'm a classic condition type II in Pete's first book. After I became semi wheel chair immobile this past summer, I finally cracked the book open in desperation June, 2015 for the first time. Far too late. From June to September 15, without fail, I performed the daily stretching routine and also re-read both books multiple times. None of it did my troubled knee any good. However all my joints quit clicking for the first time in my life and the obvious foot eversion disappeared quickly. My hips started swinging for the first time ever and I began walking down the stairs feet pointed straight ahead. That was all good, but the knee cartilage had deteriorated too far. It was too late. I was at the end of the line and knew it was time to visit my long time Trusted California Chiropractic Doctors for some critical consultation. That happened mid-September, 2015.

Little did I know that many years ago one of these very same Doctors had personally worked and studied with Pete in his San Diego clinic a few hours per week. I never knew.

Here is how he became a believer in this obscure ex Vietnam Vet turned magic healer. Pete's office was literally just upstairs from this Doctor's office. This Chiropractor would see people hobble past his office, climb up a set of stairs and sometime later, fluidly walk back out the door. That got his attention. He thought, "Who is this guy upstairs without a professional Dr. Shingle on his door?" From those very early days many years ago, my Chiropractic Doctor friend has never stopped recommending Pete's methods to stay pain free. After you read his book, it'll make crystal clear sense why there's an epidemic of joint deterioration and joint pain going on in the United States.

In a nutshell, Pete has shown us without doubt, that if our walking gait is compromised for whatever reason, it shows up very obviously in our posture. Foot eversions and pronations are a dead giveaway that a person is heading for some type of joint pain and serious malady in their lifetime. Even just one foot, very slightly everted, will affect everything from a golf swing, to dance steps, to standing in line at the grocery store, and can be structurally linked up into the ankles, knees, hips, spine, elbows, shoulders and even up to the neck and skull and will most likely eventually cause big trouble. Straighten up everted feet and our posture improves markedly, our hips begin to swing naturally and we walk with more authority and natural sexiness. We look nicer, act sexier and our golf swing can finally begin to improve. There's a lot more to it but that's my short version. Read the book and you get it all.

Who would've thought that walking very slightly duck footed could ruin our joints and put us in the hospital for surgery twenty years later. I'm proof positive. Next time you're in the shopping mall notice the high percentage of people who have at least one foot slightly pointed outward as they walk. It's epidemic and so is joint pain. It's everywhere all the time. It's so subtle that virtually nobody knows if they walk that way or not. If those feet of ours aren't lined up and walking dead straight ahead . . . big trouble lies ahead. Can you imagine driving a car for 20 years with the front right wheel toed outward 10 or 15 degrees? The cars' tires would constantly be scrubbing off. Can you imagine the constant torque placed on the front ball joints in such a misaligned car suspension? Our human joints get crucified with this type of misalignment and we ignore it every day of our life. His book goes into all this. Once you see his diagrams and explanations it's all very obvious. Bottom line, deal with it now, or wind up like me. His books are a great start for understanding the problem and getting a stretching routine introduced into your overall health plan.

My 1st Recommendation:
The Egoscue Method of Health Through Motion: Revolutionary Program That Lets You Rediscover the Body's Power to Rejuvenate It, by Pete Egoscue (amazon.com)

My 2nd Recommendation:
Pain Free: A Revolutionary Method for Stopping Chronic Pain, by Pete Egoscue (amazon.com)

My Grandma Told Me So

Today at my age, I remember precious few words that my grandmother ever said to me, mostly because the fog of time has rolled in heavy after 63 years, but these three phrases she spoke directly to me do remain in my mind very clearly today. Interesting how the mind filters, imprints or discards a lifetime of sensory input. She said these three magic things to me before age ten, over fifty years ago: *"Jimmy Jam, your health is the most important thing you will ever have, take care of it." "Good beds and good shoes will give you a good life." "Buy the best furniture once, and it will last you a lifetime like this chair."*

Pretty interesting last comment to a pre-teen, but understandable if you knew my grandmother. I remember that chair to this day: It had bold lion heads carved into the ends of its polished hardwood armrests. She was of solid German stock, her family had emigrated a generation before to America, she a nurse, her spouse, a no nonsense German architect of note. If nothing else, they were model grandparents of complete practicality and wanted nothing less than German efficiency for their offspring. Her words found a home with me. Her advice about beds came into serious consideration by necessity after back surgery at a young age. Today I have no qualms about rejecting a hotel room if the bed isn't suitable. I'll drive an extra twenty miles if necessary to look after my back because I can spot a bad bed from 600 yards, hanging upside down from a tree, blindfolded, in the rain, and intoxicated. I know beds.

As far as furniture, that directive came into play once we could afford long-lived furniture. My grandma would be proud of our comfortable household. In fact we try to purchase everything *once and done.*

As far as good shoes? Well for 63 years and 7 1/2 months, I thought I knew a thing or two about good shoes. My confirmation bias was my eternal guide. I always found if they fit well, were well constructed and durable, looked good and were the top recommended brand name, my feet were well served. Twenty years ago, a climbing boot specialist suggested I add in a thirty-dollar pair of inserts to the purchase. "No, I've been fine without them all my life. I don't have fallen arches." I said. I didn't know what I didn't know!

This is leading right to your tired misaligned feet, Dear Reader, and this is important.

When a younger man was assisting my wife push me from the SNCF, TGV underground rail platform at Charles De Gaulle Airport in Pairs back in September, up and out to the International Terminal, I struck up a conversation. I like people everywhere and always enjoy hearing the story of anybody's life journey if they have the time to share. It's just something I enjoy.

He was with us for a good half hour pushing between connections so I had time to ask him what he did when he wasn't at the airport pushing old farts like me. That kind of an open- ended question can blossom into hours for the enthusiastic storyteller. He bit the hook and was off into his private world far beyond his day job.

He was rather pleased to tell us that he ran the Paris full marathon this past spring and finished in a very respectable time. A magnificent day for everybody but particularly himself because it was his first one . . . and with a very good time. Knowing other marathoners and tri-athletes over the years, I asked him how many years had he trained. He told us *forever*.

By now, my wife was also intrigued by this young man's passion to hear the rest of his story. He explained that up until this early spring before the marathon, he could never run more than four to six miles. He said his ankles and knees killed him running. *Hello Jim Lindl !!!* That got my attention!

I was incredulous, and asked him how he got from 6 miles capability to 26 miles in such short order! He said his secret was because of custom shoe inserts. I further asked if that was it. And he happily confirmed that, that was it! He went on to explain about some obscure computer analysis of his feet where he stood on a box with light shining upwards and it read out how and why his feet needed leveling out to correct for arch and bone dysfunctions. He said there were only two in Paris doing this new thing, so I figured that was a dead end for me right there. I was in a wheel chair on-route to California in a few hours anyway. We got to the end of my push ride and he disappeared to help the next person in need of a ride. I never found out from him who provided his magic Parisian marathon inserts but I sure wanted to find out more after hearing his story . . . and I eventually did.

A day later, while sitting in an office familiar to me for the past ten years, sat a metal box, on the floor, beside a Chiropractors desk. I paid no attention to it. I had traveled 31 hours to get my neck adjusted by a trusted specialist, not look at a metal box on his clinic floor. Now understand this is a pretty special doctor I purposely traveled to see. After using chiropractors for now 44 years, I've a keen appreciation for the difference range of ability from average to the extraordinary, to the very rare gifted ones. He's a very rare gifted one. Not only is he the magic Doctor for my neck treatment, but he's a professional golfer, and a seriously good guitar picker and vocalist. I've never seen him on the course but I've heard him crooning down at the coffee shop. This is probably one of the most accomplished two legged beings I've ever met. Besides that, he's a genuinely nice all around guy. He's the same Doctor that pressed Pete Egoscue's book into my hands ten years ago which I never read.

On his floor was a machine just like the one in Paris that the wheel chair man talked about that reads feet . . . but it didn't register with me. My doctor wasn't talking about it, and it never dawned on me to ask him what this box was all about until my wife walked into the room with a stray office brochure, and exclaimed, "Jim, I've found those shoe inserts the guy in Paris was talking about." "Where?" I asked. "Right here!" she said.

Hiding in plain sight but once again, either ignored or dismissed in my subconscious biases. James Redfield, in his classic book *Celestine Prophecy*, suggests through his beautifully told story, that unseen forces or spirit guides are out there trying to help us poor, earthling imbeciles from stumbling through life, but, we have to do our part of one important thing: Pay attention to the messages, signals, and signs presented before us as we journey through life. There's no doubt in my mind during this time of deep need, things were put out for me to pick up and interpret. The wheel chair guy was a messenger of help more than appreciated at the time. Somebody knew I was going directly toward that obscure machine that I thought, "I'm never going to find."

Well this is a lot of keystrokes burnt up telling a story for what. The proof is in the pudding I say. I got my feet read by the light-box, and after returning home received the custom-built orthotics that cost a pretty penny. Were these shoe inserts going to do any good considering my worn out joint condition? I'd soon find out.

I mentioned earlier that I did fourteen straight weeks, June to September 15, 2015 every single day, of Egoscue's condition II full stretching routine. That should have been enough to straighten out a pretzel and it did, except for a lazy left foot that was folded inward underneath me. It was readily apparent whenever I'd lay on the bed with both feet hanging over the edge. That left foot always flopped underneath me. I called it a lazy left ankle. It's been that way for at least thirty plus years. Why I don't know. It was never injured that I recall.

I've put these magic inserts into my house slippers or my outdoor boots, whichever I'm wearing. In just over a month, that lazy bent ankle is 100% gone! Just another piece of the puzzle. Who would've thought that simple inserts could change our overall body alignment and allow us to maybe, go run a marathon? Not me before trying these inserts.

So now, you know why I spent so much time rehashing all this history on Egoscue and Foot Levelers. This young man was able to run the 2015 Paris Marathon because of the simple addition of shoe inserts. Would you buy a pair too, if you had a bum knee like mine? You'll have to answer that question yourself. Plenty of good stuff to read about shoe inserts on this site: Custom Orthotics (Foot Levelers)

If I had just recommended that you simply check the yellow pages for foot levelers or read Egoscue without all this back-story, I suspect your biases like mine, could have concluded everything for you without having a serious look. The take away is this: If it's good enough for Jack Nicklaus or worked for a public caregiver who out ran forty thousand others in his first Paris Marathon, I believe it's worth a person's consideration before they wind up with a bum knee like mine.

Authorship & Authority

Whenever I read anything of critical importance, I like to know who the author is. The root of the word author stems from the word authority. I always want to know the authors' authority, and if possible, glean their core philosophies within their subject exposed, their integrity, and their sincerity before I invest too much time listening to or reading their message. I think it's very important for readers to expect the author to earn the readers trust as a book's pages progress. Maybe it can happen very quickly if a powerful celebrity endorses a person. Maybe we trust something because it's on the bestseller list or it's the latest buzzy trend of the Internet.

For me, I want to earn your careful attention to this book by the truth of my story that's gradually unfolding as I write. I believe true authorship is an earned right. Authority isn't validated just because a person's name is on a book.

A Little Bit Of Background On Me

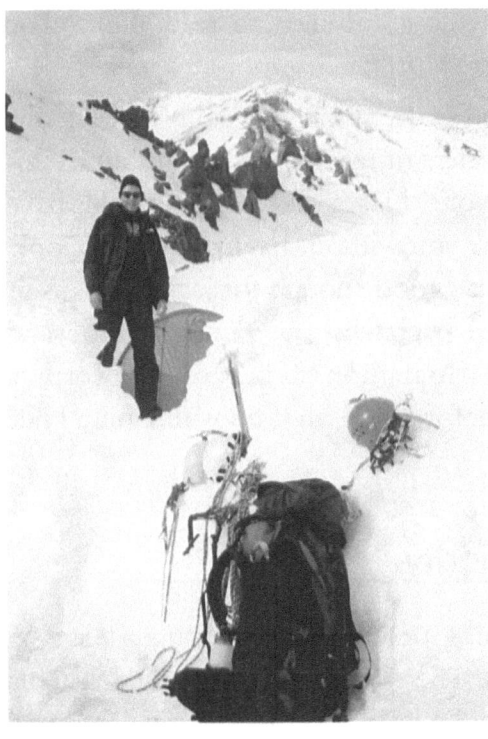

Mount Shasta, California
Casaval Ridge
April, 2004
© 2016 Jim Lindl

Dug-in, wind-protected high camp at 10,300 feet elevation at the top end of Giddy-Giddy Gulch. The summit in the clouds is about four miles away at 14,179-foot elevation. The lenticular cloud formation indicates potential high winds on the summit. The alpine packs, climbing gear, and ropes clock in at 65 pounds each. I didn't have a hint of sore knees in this picture at 52 years of age. Just some clicking in one hip and both knees.

Three years later, in 2007, I retired from my involved US business and became a simple French gardener on our 8-acre farm in Dordogne, France. I can't believe how my health deteriorated in only 11 short years.

Back in the day, Mount Shasta was one of my favorite early spring training grounds for serious more difficult climbs later each season. I climbed this mountain by various routes 12 different times in four years. This was a trip guiding two friends. This midrange technical route is never crowded. You can read more about Casaval here. It's a beautiful airy line to the top of Misery Hill, then on to the summit pinnacle. Mt. Shasta Casaval Ridge (Mt. Shasta Avalanche Center)

At that age, I had a powerful sustained mountaineer's endurance and deep reservoirs of will power that non-alpinists could never begin to understand. It was built up over years of disciplined outdoor activity that started early on in my days as a young, west coast, old growth timber faller. At the time of that mountain picture, I was a model of health and fitness and totally pain free. I ate very carefully, avoided alcohol, supplemented with the best vitamins on the planet, and lived a successful stress free business executive life with ample free time to travel and climb year round.

Today, eleven short years later I now need a wheel chair to get across an international airport or I could never make the connections. I'd need to crawl on the floor of the airport to get from one end to the other. I lack the strength and endurance to walk more than three hundred yards as I sit in this chair today. I sit here typing and wondering, "what happened". I think I know the whole picture as I write this book today . . . but six months ago, I didn't have a clue about Lyme disease or that I had its symptoms in triple full house spades.

I tell you this part of my history to have you get a feel how fast a person's health can collapse. Did I need Pete Egoscue's stretching back then? Most assuredly. *I didn't know what I didn't know.* A year after this picture was taken, I received Pete's book but it was never read until last June, ten years too late.

For the past 42 years my health maintenance bias was exclusively tuned into Chiropractors and then, for the past 23 years, additionally tuned into my company's vitamins and clean healthy living. I believed that was enough. Chiropractic adjustments on my Neck and Back and a careful clean lifestyle allowed me to build up good fundamental core health to live an active life as you can see in the picture.

My *bias* was simple: Neck and Back, Chiropractic treatment, clean balanced living and vitamins . . . for decades. That's what I knew and it worked pretty well . . . until it didn't.

Chiropractic care became my vital lifeline after a very early age back surgery. The surgical MDs said they could do no more for me, except continue prescribing more painkillers once their surgery was completed two hours later. They went as far as they could go on my back and when I walked out that University of Alberta hospital door Christmas Eve, 1976, I was on my own and knew it. I had been on Valium for over ten weeks waiting for surgery and I felt deeply depressed. I felt lower than low for the first time in my life. I flushed hundreds of Valium pills down the toilet that Christmas day. Several huge bottles full of them. When a logger is all busted up and washed up, they say in the woods: "He's run out of timber", and I did at age 24.

I was physically spent and emotionally alone in my apartment that Christmas Eve day. I knew I needed to change. I needed to set a new sail physically, mentally, emotionally, financially, spiritually, and socially . . . and I eventually did. That transition was the darkest and hardest period of my entire life until today. I feel like I'm there again at age 63, but unlike age 24, on the down slope side of my life.

For all those years since then, because of my deeply ingrained confirming biases toward chiropractors, I was tuned out and turned off to just about anything else. That was my bias, unfortunately for me, even though I very well knew, there's always more out there, if we keep our minds open. It is just plain hard to think outside of our self-imposed box. I felt safe and secure marching to my long time familiar drummers.

Do I think today that the Egoscue method would've made a difference? Absolutely. Do I still think I needed all those Chiropractors back in the day? Absolutely. I'd probably be dead and gone without them. My back surgery was just a crisis stopgap measure that allowed me to transition from literally crawling around my apartment floor in December 1976, at age 24 to walking again. So yes, the surgery too, was vital. However, I don't believe any one modality is the total magic bullet. I think we have to find a blend of healing modalities to achieve optimal sustained holistic health. That's what I'm trying to point out from my experience at 63 years of age.

Chiropractors have provided critical spinal and neck adjustments on me over the past four decades and have been indispensable in my life functioning. But not once did they look at my walking gait or suggest I could be looking at trouble with my knees. One tried educating me by gifting Pete's book, but unfortunately, I never read it. That's the message of my story here. This isn't criticism. This is awareness for everybody, Patients and Doctors alike. We're all in this great whirl and mystery of life together.

How The Lyme Picture Came Into Focus

I was bitten just one single time by a tick in Fall 2007 here in France. What type, I don't know. We have eight acres of beautiful rich bottom land with a nice small bog and wild flower meadow, a small forest, three hundred meters of river frontage and magnificent organic gardens. This is old rural France at its best where we're surrounded by rolling forested hills, small farms and nice quiet country people.

I remember the bite distinctly because it was the first and only time in my life. I had forgotten about it entirely after an ensuing blood test indicated Lyme negative. I never gave Lyme another thought for seven years. The tick bit me on the right knee, left-hand quarter just above the kneecap. That same knee is the candidate for double amputation, which is necessary for an artificial knee joint to be inserted. Is there a correlation between Lyme infection and my knee deterioration? Who knows for sure. I think there's a strong probability because of the speed of cartilage deterioration and the history of knee pain right after the tick bite.

The initial mild Lyme symptoms cropped up shortly after the bite. I didn't make the correlation. I was busy gardening and living a simple clean healthy rural French lifestyle. Later, other and progressively worse ones joined these very same symptoms until they eventually steamrolled over me to today's debilitating mess. Yet as good as the French Health system is, at the time, they dismissed any notion of Lyme disease because of my negative blood work and otherwise outward appearance of strong health. I find all this incredulous today; knowing what I now know about Lyme disease, because we live in one the most tick infested Lyme regions in all of Europe! Limoges, France is noted for its

Lyme Medical expertise, and this major city is only sixty miles from our farm, and all my doctors here have access to them. Yet the blood labs and the local Doctors dismissed the possibility of Lyme Malady entirely back then, seven years ago.

Thanks to Dr. Halverstadt's extremely detailed examination methods plus some of his patient and colleagues' direct experience with Lyme, did I finally learn what was very probably killing all my joints. He's the second Chiropractic Doctor we had scheduled during our California medical trip.

He quickly zeroed in on the Medical System's "taboo" subject, of Lyme disease. He enlightened me of that possibility given my obvious multiple Lyme symptoms. I had never considered Lyme before Mid-September, 2015 until I visited him in California. He's an extremely trusted chiropractor. I've known David for years because of some alternative treatments he had done for both me my wife. He's a professional colleague of the guitar picking Chiropractor and both of them knew I was coming to town in a wheel chair.

I had numerous classic symptoms he identified as Lyme indicators: Heart palpitation, shortness of breath, lightening eye flashes, hot inflamed knee joint, depression, fuzzy thinking, chronic fatigue and on and on . . . I could barely walk a hundred yards, but never related it to a resident bacterial infection in my joints. During his examination, I failed to remember that singular tick bite from seven years before. It was totally outside of my current consciousness and never mentioned it to him, until he said it looks like you have Lyme symptoms to me and explained how a Lyme bacterial infection lies hidden and hard to detect. Bingo!

It all became crystal clear in an instant. It all made sense to me from that day forward. I could now visualize those nasty looking corkscrew-like spirochete bacteria burrowing under my kneecaps into deep tissue. Up to that point, I thought I was just an old, broken down genetically deficient short-timer with no hope. I told this Doctor as much: "I feel old and atrophied." I told him. He said, "You are *not* old." I said, "Yes I am." And out the door I went.

Every proper three-act novel or movie has its catalyst, its spark, that iconic action scene or dramatic dialogue that gets the whole show on the road at the beginning of the first act. It's called "The inciting incident". Now Jim Lindl had his inciting incident. He was presented with his personal enemy to fight. The question was how? That fateful day in San Luis Obispo in Doctor Halverstadt's office was my *eureka* moment. That appointment which required 31 hard hours of international travel was a pivotal moment for the rest of my life. That appointment was the inciting incident that forever changed the direction in my life because I now had a real live enemy to fight. I knew I'd figure it out somehow and dig myself out of this deep depressing dark hole within which I was trapped.

Dr. Halverstadt is the quiet unsung hero in my life. He's a gifted healer and a special type of chiropractor with unusual dedication. A compassionate, gentle man and a relentless seeker of better health through his profession. He, to me, identified the root cause of my collapsing health. But he too doesn't have all the answers. He admitted as much in his office that day. His field is primarily structural alignment, and although he suspected what was eating me up inside, he didn't have a definitive solution for my Lyme problem. He made that very clear to me. That would have to come later through more research on my part. He did assure me though, Lyme bacteria are tough nasty bastards to kill off.

Others would have to join this story later to provide the path out of my dark swamp of distress. His clinical examination of my exasperating condition that September day, is the inciting incident to this whole story. Without him, I wouldn't be writing this today. I would've continued with my downward spiral into darkness, wondering why I was so physically weak, mentally tired and lacked motivation and mental focus with creeping episodes of depression.

We all need to keep an open mind and understand that there are numerous factors we need to consider when tackling a problem. None of us singularly has all the answers, but together we can put our heads together for better living.

Here is an acronym I've used and taught for years:

T E A M: Together, Everybody, Achieves, More.

Doctor Halverstadt is the first person I want to thank publicly in this Book.

Chapter 2:
Pills, Potions, Lotions & Other Sundry Concoctions In a Bottle

Since Mach 17, 1993, I've had an extraordinary bias toward vitamin supplementation. One company in particular . . . the one that I helped found and was my business for over twenty years. It used to be my 24/7 life passion and my vision for a better future. Our young California Company quietly cut a wide swath across America for one simple reason: We had science- based leading edge products that worked better than anything on the planet at the time. We were absolutely better than anything on the market, anywhere worldwide. Our business growth model was very easy back then because there were few effective alternatives if a person wanted products that delivered real measurable results. Nutritional supplementation hadn't gone mainstream yet. GMO crop production and general public knowledge of the hideous factory produced food chain was in its infancy. A meat and potatoes diet with a few veggies thrown in was an acceptable eating standard for most in that generation. Little did Americans want to believe back then that we were slowly killing ourselves with expensive hollow poisoned food from farm field to the table.

Today, when I leave Europe and land at any major American Airport, the state of American health is immediately apparent. It's deplorable and it shows in the public waistline and the cost of medical care. What our vitamin company forecasted, what was going to happen to America's health, 23 years ago when I helped found that company in March of 1993, has arrived . . . almost to the state of near total health chaos. Vast swaths of humanity are today grappling with that reality and seeking sustainable solutions to ensure their personal health security. It's a very big deal with solutions hiding in plain sight, in my opinion.

Our main vitamin competition back then was grocery store chewables. The plethora of alternatives we have today was just beginning to arrive over the horizon. Our company believed we had a wide-open field to ourselves because of our incredible customer results that ensured their loyalty to always come back to us first . . . and they did. All the later-day brand name energy drinks that rolled across America in the late 90's and beyond, were still in the competitors' laboratories, while our magic potions were solving the conundrum of adolescent and adult ADD/ADHD by the droves all across America. Migraine headaches, skin disorders, chronic fatigue, and all kinds of general malaise were almost miraculously banished with the use of our products. Not occasionally, but almost 100% of the time. We witnessed firsthand how vital the connection is between complete absorbable nutrition and sound vital health across thousands and thousands of customers nationwide. Who would've thought that our food supply was killing us. We at our company knew, while the *Fast Food Nation* ate its way into deeper sickness.

The mainstream food supply has become terribly deficient and over processed. Since I've retired from that realm, it has only gotten more challenging to find good clean affordable non-GMO food in America. It's one of the reasons we retired to France, bought 8 acres of pristine bottomland and turned it into an organic veggie farm. GMO in the food supply is totally banned across Europe as well as the use of stimulative growth hormones and antibiotics in animal feed chop.

Four hundred and fifty million Europeans and an additional 150 million Russians all get along fine without GMO crops and these six hundred million people have no trouble feeding themselves affordable healthy food. You ask how do they keep GMO crop production out of Europe.

Have a look at a typical French farmer protest. It's not unusual that they express democracy in France this vocally. You may think it's extreme, but it works. Protesting French Farmers Dump & Spray . . . Gov't Buildings, November 05, 2014 (YouTube) and French Farmers Stage Tractor Protest In Paris, France 24, September 03, 2015 and World's Largest Country, Russia, Bans GMO Food Crops, Mint Press News, October 05, 2015

The French don't vote just once every four years. They vote on the streets with their protests regularly. These *manifestations* are more like street plebiscites than a protest. Protest is culturally imbedded here since the revolution over two hundred years ago and they've never stopped fighting for their rights.

It's part of their national way of life and very different from the United States these days. Everyday ordinary people are never afraid to speak up vigorously to express their opinions in France. It's what keeps Paris cafes always humming.

Back To The Vitamins

In a nutshell, our vitamin products were absorbable at a deep cellular level, and when the body is well nourished, it repairs itself. Our products did exactly that. It was a patented process that made our products effective, and unique.

I crisscrossed the United States for four glorious start-up years spreading the word, sometimes teamed up with lecturing physicians and brilliant scientists who saw the light, and also championed our products from the podium of conference halls. They validated with science the truth behind our magic powders and potions and it all made irrefutable sense to everybody simply because our customers got stellar results.

Even the scientists who formulated and bottled our potions were sometimes surprised how well the body will heal itself if the right nutrition is in place and can be absorbed. It happened thousands and thousands of times to new customers every year. It was a sight to behold.

One of those Doctors I traveled with on our lecture circuit was a noted MD, author and lecturer, who was classically trained and practiced traditional medicine in the US Medical system for years. He eventually crossed the Rubicon from traditional Allopathic medicine over to the Ayurvedic and holistic medical realm and stayed in that camp for good. Among his patients was Sylvester Stallone along with a bevy of other Hollywood notables. One of this Doctor's claims to fame is that back in the day, he had treated over ten thousand patients without using a single prescription drug. He lectured the public that our company's vitamins worked so miraculously because of our patented absorption technology. That was evident to everybody because of the simple fact they worked so well . . . That's why he lectured for our company.

I tell you all this back-story to give you an idea of the companions I used to tag along with on a lecture circuit. I can talk a good game not because I'm scientifically educated.

Quite the contrary. It's partially because for an important formative period of time, I listened to and studied some of the best in the world and some of *their* brilliance got infused into my brain and some of it stuck. I've always appreciated good science . . . and science fiction, which often is foisted off as truth. History tells us modern dogmatic science is often only the partial truth but not the whole truth under the sun. It' up to us to distill the difference and it's not easy.

Was I biased against other nutritional products? Of course. I was so confident in our leading edge products and our stellar customer track record that I always told our field of distributors that if they could ever find anything better, they should distribute them . . . not ours. I always told them, "Your health is more important than your money."

Along with two venture capitalists, I was the founding Executive director of that company and responsible for the creation of our entire fifty statewide distribution network that eventually grew into hundreds of thousands of happy loyal customers that bought from us with industry beating loyalty. Tens upon tens of Millions of dollars' worth of products went through our distribution channels. The name of the company isn't important. It's just a footnote in the dustbin of business history today twenty-three years after I helped open the doors.

That company changed hands through a series of different owners and in an increasingly heavily populated and sophisticated vitamin marketplace with rapidly improving products; they were eventually forced to shutter their doors. Thankfully, all the products live on and the legacy of our customers' excellence continues in the company that bought us out. It was a good time for me to retire and move on . . . and I did.

Why do I tell you all this? Because there was a very important intersection of all this background, hiding right square in front of my nose that I missed completely. Are my magic vitamins the complete nutritional answer for the human body? I used to think so up until I couldn't walk any longer and I was forced to go beyond my bias. I had to get my head out of the sand and take a look around for alternative treatments. If ever a person had a bias toward a particular nutritional support program, it was me. And today I've paid the price for that narrow-minded focus.

Science moved on and I wasn't paying attention to the direction it headed. I became a French gardener and left myself behind the advancements in nutritional science.

As good as all my alma mater's products were they didn't grow any extra cartilage in my knees when it was needed. I still take my vitamins every single day and have since March 17, 1993, the day we opened the company doors. Am I healthier for it? Of course. Markedly so but I don't continue to take them for any hope of knee repair. However, tangentially, they did lead me to a Naturopathic Doctor who does have the answer. He has a lot of answers about a lot of important health things. He constantly lectures via his private subscription-based webinars on behalf of the company who bought us out two years ago; all the while, I've been a retired *Rip Van Winkle* living in France. I never bothered looking into this new parent company's research base because I was too busy raising organic vegetables in France and taking my original magic vitamins.

It was only after I put out a Lyme disease distress SOS in October, 2015 to one of my most trusted long time vitamin business colleagues in Billings, Montana. We all call her CK. She and I worked closely together in that Vitamin Company from the day we opened our doors until different owners took over the wheel, who then went on and eventually shuttered the doors for good.

She alerted me to a noted lecturer and healer named Doctor Peter Glidden. ND. CK had recently heard one of his live lectures and told me he also has a video lecture series with one of the feature presentations geared to healing Lyme disease naturally. Bingo! *Hello Jim!* This teacher Dr. Glidden had arrived and the student Jim Lindl was ready with all ears.

Doctor Glidden had beat the crap out of his own Lyme symptoms years ago and knew a ton about this disease as evidenced in his riveting 60 minute video lecture. In fact, he used to have his office just down the road from Lyme, Connecticut, the epicenter of Lyme where it was first officially identified in the 1980s. This Doctor picked up for me where Dr. Halverstadt in California left off, like a perfect baton pass in a medical relay race to a solution somewhere down the road.

Before talking to this long time Montana business colleague, I thought I had all the fundamental answers about a lot of health stuff. I wasn't interested in what the nutritional world was up to because my business was completed in that industry and I had moved on to healthier non GMO pastures in organic Old France. Thankfully, she had stayed somewhat current in the latest thinking about Lyme, while I didn't have a clue.

James Redfield with his message strikes again! If we just look around and pay attention, gifted solutions to our problems can be hiding in plain sight. CK is the second person I want to thank publicly in this book: She brought Dr. Glidden and teasel into the picture. Without this serendipitous intersection in the story, I'd still be defenseless against this dreaded disease. First, Dr. Halverstadt, then . . . CK. The billiard balls were beginning to line up but I wasn't out of the woods just yet.

Finding the Solution

The solution to my knee troubles and Lyme disease was hiding in plain sight but couldn't see it until I overcame my deeply ingrained biases.

Until the reality of a potentially botched surgery forced me to seek out and pay attention to new and better holistic solutions available elsewhere, I was unable to break free from my old paradigm. I had lived with a confirming bias for twenty-three years until just a few weeks ago.

That bias was annihilated after I listened to a lecture by this Naturopathic healer about knee surgery, cartilage regeneration, joint health and Lyme disease. It's from one of his provocative lectures that convinced me that I must postpone my surgery and give his suggestions a shot. I've seen too much good science and good nutritional holistic healing over the years to be skeptical of his message, his wisdom and his 27 years of proven clinical experience.

I heard that he was obliquely affiliated with our new parent company but never availed myself to his lecture series. I didn't need any holistic wisdom, I thought. I needed non-GMO meat, dairy, poultry and pork, plus, delicious fresh veggies and fruit from our garden in rural France.

I invite you to listen to Dr. Glidden's *Joint and Cartilage* lecture on his subscription based educational website and decide if you were in my shoes, what would you do? Would you try his protocol for 90 days? Would you postpone imminent surgery? Would you give it a shot?

Until I listened to his lecture, I understood there to be only three options:

1) Surgery for knee replacement
2) Adult Stem Cell Treatment (possibly effective)
3) Brood, suffer and swallow painkillers

If you follow my journey in this book, you'll learn step by step how it all unfolded for me. I'm about to begin his combination protocol for both Lyme disease and cartilage rebuilding next week.

That's what this book is all about: Kicking the Lyme symptoms out of my body with an herbal regime (phytotherapy) and rebuilding my knee cartilage with a nutritional holistic protocol for the next 90 days.

So strap in and study his educational videos. Be prepared to possibly become mentally entangled, irreverently lectured, rudely shocked, irritated, sometimes agog, more than skeptical or a myriad of other deep feelings depending on your own personal biases toward doctors and healing. His lectures may rattle your chain, but you'll become better educated in the process.

He has a twenty dollar monthly subscription fee to gain access to this archive of naturopathic video lectures. It can be canceled at any time. Glidden Healthcare Advocate Info

Chapter 03:
Pulp Fiction

Sunday Night, November 29, 2015
US Thanksgiving Weekend
17 Days Until My Périgueux Surgeon's Appointment

If you watched the video lecture, you know the immediate direction I'm headed.

I'm drumming my fingers here on this computer desk tonight watching some postal tracking numbers connected to my future. These codes are attached to three heavy boxes that contain roughly a month's supply of the suggested healing protocol to rebuild my knee. They're at least a week away because they got stuck in Billings during the holiday crush and a snowstorm. CK has become my supplier who acquires everything via the Internet and transships everything over to France. It pays to have long time trusted friends in time of need.

I get the Teasel Elixir from a Teasel specialist company out of Germany. It's through them I found Dr. Storl's book on Teasel and Lyme disease that you'll hear much more about later.

Neither you nor I nor anybody else on the planet can predict how the story is going to unfold on these pages. It's a mystery to all of us from here on out. Although I've got a head start on you by watching the video and reading some books a few days before you, I feel we're both in this journey together side by side from here to the end. It's new territory for me too.

Until the products arrive, there's not much point in talking about them. When they do get here, I'll take a photo, include it with the text, and link you to more than you probably want to read. But at least you'll get a visual idea what close to five hundred bucks buys these days. I'm wondering if I can choke down all the stuff on a daily basis. It's a lot to swallow, literally.

And remember I'm an ex-vitamin guru who doesn't need to be born again to appreciate advanced scientific nutrition and supplementation. It's been an important part of my life for decades now. But even for me, I'm still from Missouri on this new option. I'm that way by nature . . . optimistic but realistic about most everything.

So what are we going to occupy ourselves with until the pills and potions arrive to activate this adult science-fair experiment? . . . how about some pulp fiction.

The balance of this chapter is pure decoration and entertainment to kill time. Like one of my mentors taught many years ago. *A stale crust of bread thrown into a dumpster might do somebody some good, even if it's just a rat or a raven.* That was probably his folksy way or rendering Shakespeare's "ill wind" mussing. Maybe something in the balance of this third chapter of rambling will benefit somebody out there who needs to experience an old crust about long ago magnificent virgin forests.

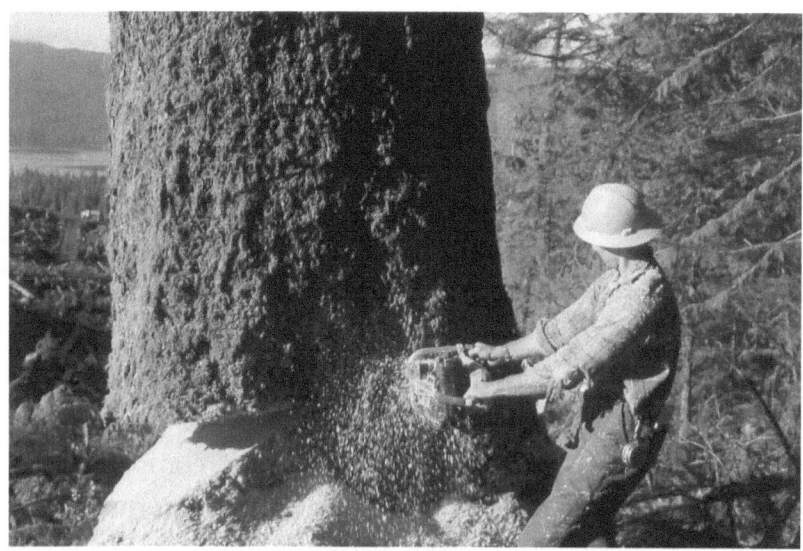

Queen Charlotte Archipelago, British Columbia, Canada
August, 1976, Jim Lindl, Timber Faller, at age 24. © 2016 Jim Lindl

600-Year-Old Growth Sitka Spruce being felled. Private operation. One hundred and ten man logging camp accessed exclusively by floatplane and tugboat barges. Relentless daily operation 6 days per week, year round, clear cutting uncountable mountain ranges from valley floors to tops of all flanking ridges. Located 90 miles offshore from Mainland B.C. and soaked with over 200 inches of annual precipitation. It's mostly all gone today except for a few parks and preservation lands, courageously saved by the First Nation with hard fought aboriginal land claims. Four months after this picture, I went through major back surgery, never to work again as a timber faller. Salt chuck in background is the ocean transport destination of this tree, before going on to worldwide pulp markets.

The Rest of the Story

I mentioned earlier that I've been fit all my life. It didn't start in the forest. It started on a farm at age 12. By age 17, I had graduated into adulthood but not high school and went directly into residency in these remote island-logging camps. I wasn't exactly raised by the wolves, but living in an isolated he-man environment for seven years is about as close as a person can get to the psychological abyss. It was a life beyond any sense of normal civilization. I loved every minute of every day of that life. It was an adventure beyond compare and it was more than a home. This type of logging environment was more akin to a holy religion. It was almost spiritual in its isolated majesty, grandeur and utter simplicity. We weren't gods, but we knew God lived among us. We were all keenly aware of our bond with something extraordinary in those magnificent isolated virgin old growth forests, far beyond the view of humanity. We may have been isolated, but we weren't alone. The spirit of those ancient trees was always present among us loggers.

I was good at cutting trees. Really good, and nicely on my way to becoming one of best. A number of kind-hearted grizzled loggers tutored a 17-year-old lost farm kid into full professional capability very quickly: I was one of their protégés. We built steep mountain access roads through impossible terrain; we charged semi-truck loads of high yield explosives down blast holes into a singular energy release that moved the unmovable. We finessed monster machinery over countless mountain ridges that lifted these whales into the salt water for delivery to far off markets. It was an incredible life for a very young man who came off a 200-acre strawberry farm.

Yes, I was fit in that day. That chainsaw in the picture had a standard short bar, 36 inches long, and with full gas and oil, it weighed in at 31 pounds. We furiously wielded those chainsaws for six hours a day like menacing light swords slicing our way through trunks and limbs, and forest debris.

For six straight hours per day, nothing could stop us. If we couldn't cut it down, then nobody else in the world could, except E.I. du Pont de Nemours and Company's high explosives. Nothing was ever left standing. We worked those tools as fast and effortlessly as a city person could swish a badminton racket.

These two-cycle McCulloch kart engines screamed 130 decibels at full wide open throttle, turning 12,000 rpm next to our face for six straight hours every single day, six days per week, year round, as long as the snow didn't get too deep. Those overstressed finely tuned saws lasted at most six months until they either seized up, blew up or got crushed by falling debris in a dangerous jackpot collapse. No ear plugs, no eye protection, no gloves.

That was all before the modern era of workplace safety and sensibility. We were left on our own to rip down the forested mountainsides, tree by tree, until there was nothing left. The pay was substantial, but it was all blood money. Every last penny.

Many timber fallers never made it out of the woods without the aid of a stretcher. It's the most dangerous occupation on the planet by a country mile. I've known that firsthand. I lasted seven years before it was my turn to get crippled and break down. In this particular camp, at age 24, I was chairman of the camp safety committee and also the camp union rep for 110 hard-nosed individuals. This is the camp where I advanced my diplomatic skills as occasional peacemaker between management and the crew and among the crew themselves sometimes as well.

Human beings can get pretty testy after working non-stop for four or five months in those conditions, with no TV, no Radio, no phones, no women, no nothing, but eat, sleep, and work six days per week unless shut-in by an occasional hurricane force storm. It was a rugged life. Fitting in and getting along is what created the human harmony in those camps. Massive amounts of timber hit the salt chuck day after day because of a highly choreographed team-based operation.

I never drank alcohol in camp so I was always reliable and careful. My character was considered trustworthy and was a notable comer . . . I got a glimpse of a woman one time in camp walking out of the engineering and planning office. She was the only female I ever saw in that logging camp. It wasn't a place for any woman. She was there no more than two hours before a floatplane gave her a ride off the island.

And Then It All Ended

Four months after that picture was taken, I crawled across my apartment floor on the 17th level of a high-rise residence in Edmonton, Alberta to dial up the neurosurgeons office for admittance into the hospital six days before Christmas. I couldn't get up off the floor to move. The doctors all told me I'd know when it was time to go under the knife and that day they agreed with me . . . it was time.

The hospital staff sent some people over to fetch me. The University Hospital was just across the street and I was so crippled up I couldn't make it there on my own steam. I stared at that hospital out of my apartment window for three long months waiting for surgery and thinking about my future. Dr.

Peter Allen a storied Canadian neurosurgeon was waiting for me, and I was ready.

Time For Change

That little episode forced me to change the direction of life. I tried going back to the woods the following spring but that first day I fired up a chainsaw and plunged it into a tree . . . well, it felt like barbed wire was being raked up and down through my spinal column. At that moment I knew I was washed up for logging and a pathetic mess at age 25 with no direction to turn. That's just about how I felt this past summer again, at age 63, when I couldn't chase the birdie a single step in our garden. Pathetically helpless with nowhere to turn.

So, Dear Reader, what's my point of all this? I simply want to make the best choices and right now, surgery for my knee is off the table if there's another solution.

Since that early back surgery there's been a lifetime of interesting twists and turns to arrive at this computer screen sitting in front of me. I offer this brief bit of back-story to simply be infused with the readers overall understanding of the following chapters as they unfold.

A few more pictures below to end this pulp fiction chapter. (*Pulp Fiction*, as in paper pulp fiction) After this editorial below, if you saw the movie, you'll understand the reason for this chapter's moniker

A Jim Lindl Chest Thumping Editorial

Here is my one and final comment for those who may criticize us for clear-cutting all those magnificent forests.

Pulp products where the destiny for the majority of all

those magnificent Q.C.I. trees: Pulp paper products like disposable tissues, absorbable cloth wipes and disposable diapers, never recycled but either flushed down the septic system or dumped into municipal landfills. If everybody in the western world would just have quit wiping with toilet paper like the other half of the world, and used machine-washed traditional cloth baby diapers like the old days, we loggers could've gone home and left those monarchs standing in peace.

Life, like war, is more complicated than emotional sound bites and photo ops on TV. I wish there was a better way, a different way. Today, I feel like we were sociopaths demolishing an ancient Spiritual Cathedral never to be re-built for another 600 years. Today I feel like that logging life was some bizarre violent fictional movie. Like a pulp fiction movie.

Some people feel that way about our modern factory food production methods, our over stressed ground water supply and the chaotic American health care system today. Unfortunately, the cathedral we are now destroying is our own body.

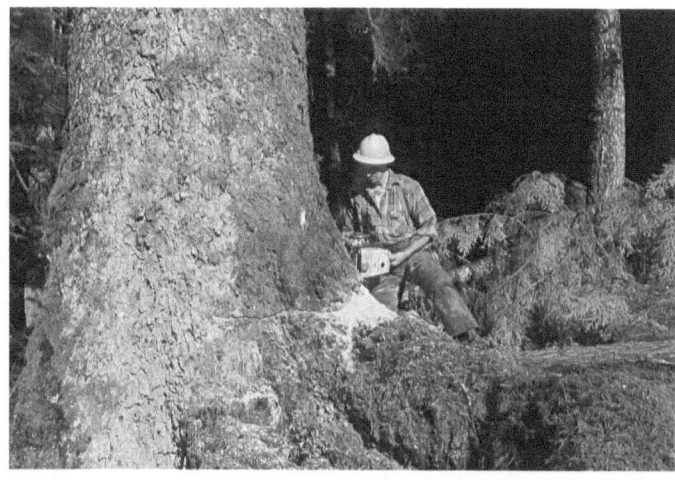

Placing the first directional cut into a 7-foot diameter Sitka Spruce Stump. Small Hemlock trees in background were nipped off in preparation. © 2016 Jim Lindl

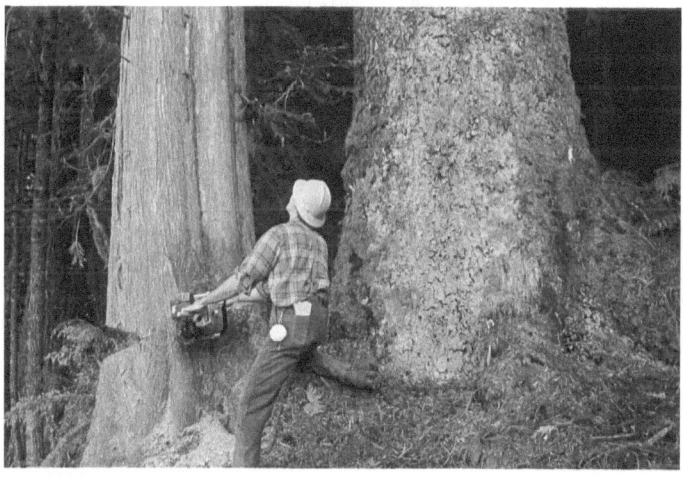

This young Western Red Cedar was pre-cleared to allow room for the Sitka Spruce. Clear knot free Cedar is a premium lumber material used for sauna paneling, home siding and roofing shingles. Each tree extremely valuable. This cedar was felled and bucked into logs lengths in less than 10 minutes. Many ancient Old Growth Cedars on this island were over 1,000 year old and 10 feet in diameter. They're virtually all gone. © 2016 Jim Lindl

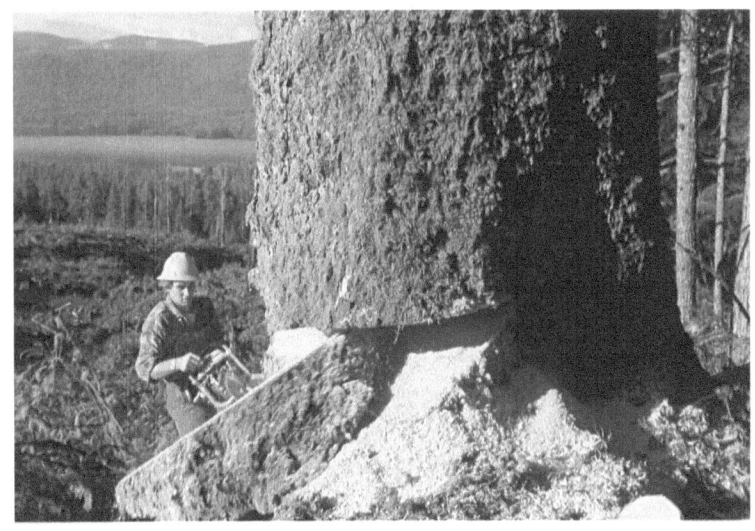

Everything is ready for the final back cut, a salt-water bay in background. This is considered an easy tree, on easy terrain. © 2016 Jim Lindl

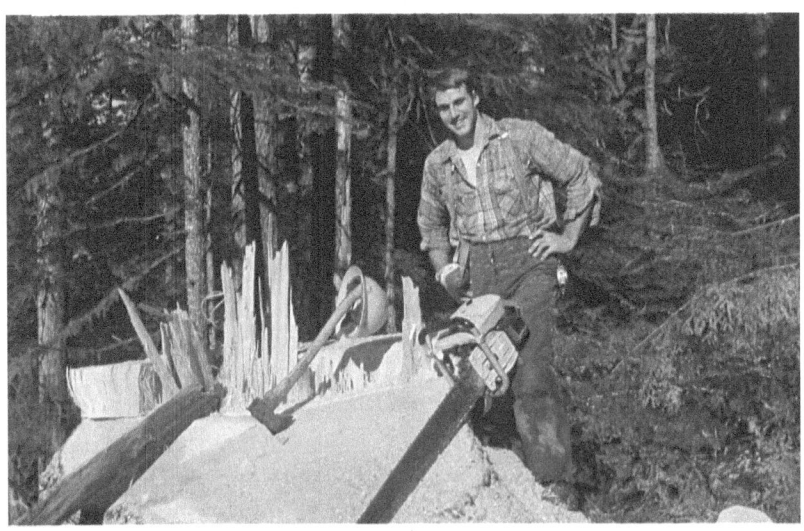

Clean safe Sitka Spruce stump. Total time for this first procedure was 20 minutes. Saw is a 125cc McCulloch sp125, .404 chisel bit, hand filed & semi-skip chain. A rare sunny day on the Islands. © 2016 Jim Lindl

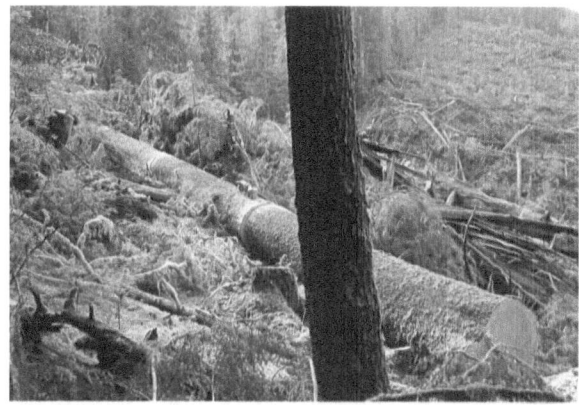

An average Sitka Spruce, about 200,000 pounds total weight. 18,120 board feet of clear perfect wood. Log specs: (34' by 65", 40' by 55", 40' by 45", 40' by 32"). 154 feet of cut logs. The top was trashed to splinters. Total tree height over 200 feet. 45 minutes to cut into lengths. This was considered easy ground to fell timber. Notice smashed rotten cedar downhill. © 2016 Jim Lindl

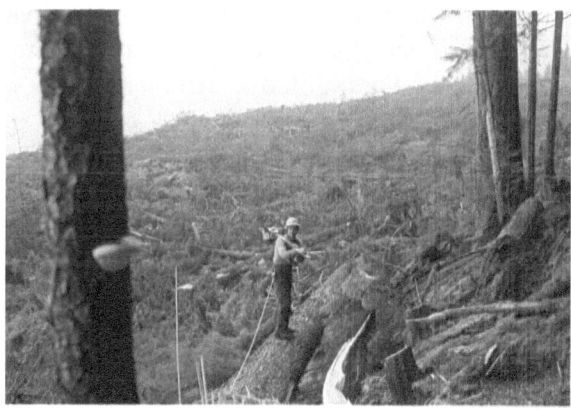

Typical clear-cut operation on the Queen Charlotte Islands. Many of these Ancient Forest Giants were considered commercially useless, were culled out & stayed in the forest to rot. British Columbia has tens of thousands of square miles stripped like this. I was one of over 2,000 fallers and part of that process for 7 years on the BC Coast. One tree at a time. 50 men with chainsaws could knock down an entire mountain range in a few years' time. My employer had 600 of them, and we were never out of work. © 2016 Jim Lindl

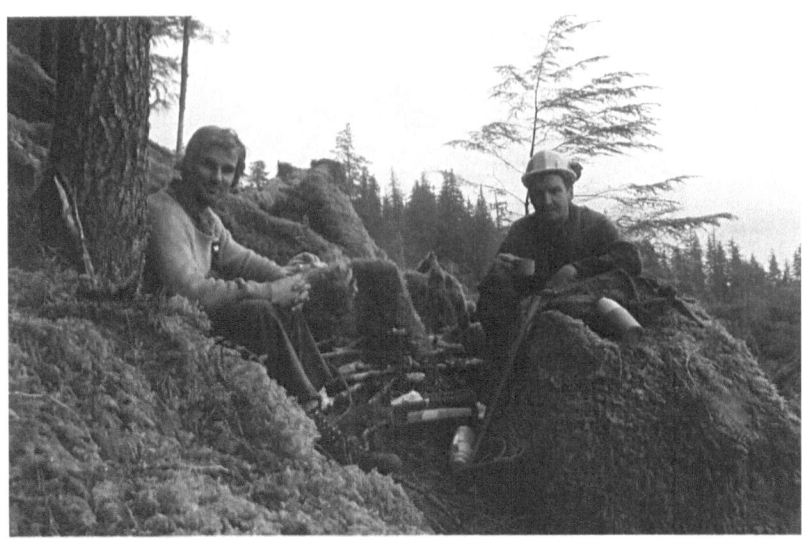

Typical noon lunch fire. My cutting partner and I were on this mountainside for a few months of clear cutting. This timber face we were opening was a half-mile long. The timber seemed endless. He sang beautiful Ukrainian melodies all day long while working. Notice I'm wearing a heavy wool top in August. In constant rainy drizzly weather, wool kept us warm in those mountains. This west coast mountain range receives over 200 inches of rain per year. These islands are about one quarter the size of Switzerland. We cut everything in sight until the Native Indians Land Claims stopped the logging. The majority of these islands were cut and leveled by pairs of timber cutters. Like what you see here. © 2016 Jim Lindl

Chapter 4:
Weeds In The Ditch

Tuesday, December 01, 2015
15 Days To Périgueux Surgeon's Appointment

This chapter isn't for the squeamish. This chapter is primarily about Lyme disease, also called by some experts, "Deer Syphilis". It's called that because deer carry it, then ticks bite deer, and later these same ticks bite humans and it acts very much like syphilis. That's the vector. That's how the spirochete spiral Lyme bacteria attack us . . . With syphilitic like ferocity. It's very hard to detect, and very hard to kill off. It acts on the human body very similar to syphilis, maybe worse. It's one nasty bastard.

If you decide to take a pass on this chapter, do know that I offer in this chapter another even higher charged intellectual feast by Dr. Glidden. He's linked immediately below. This next provocative lecture is about Lyme disease and how to beat it holistically. Some viewers may think he gets a bit uppity, so strap in tight. He lectures at gale force intensity in parts of this one and it leads directly up to weeds growing in the ditch right in front of our next-door neighbor's cabinet shop. It's called Wild Teasel (*dipsacus sylvestris*), a very powerful and proven Lyme bacteria killer-agent according to Professor Storl. Once again a proven remedy for my problems, hiding in plain sight. Who would've known, and yet it's all explained in this insightful video lecture. My head was nicely "stuck in the sand" on this one for a second round of ignorant neglect.

To get access to the entire Glidden lecture library there's a subscription fee of 20 dollars per month. It can be cancelled at any time. It's on this site, with his Lyme lecture, that I began to find the direction out of my swamp of discontent. Glidden Healthcare Advocate Info

Dear Reader, if you have gotten this far in the journey and watched both these video lectures you have plenty to chew on for a few days.

I'll return to writing a bit later. I've got some important new reading to do. It's a book by a world authority on beating Lyme using the Teasel root. It's title, *Healing Lyme Disease Naturally*, by Dr. Wolf-Dieter Storl. He's a noted Medical Anthropologist who contracted Lyme disease and beat it with Teasel. I read his introduction and was hooked. It reads more like a mystery novel in search of the Templar's gold.

The iconic American author, teacher and world-renowned lecturer of herbal remedies, Matthew Wood, wrote this Teasel book's glowing forward to the author Dr. Storl. Wood's seminal writings are considered *the* touchstone reference of modern Herbal Medicine, worldwide. Wood is an American, who lives in the forest of Northern Wisconsin and is active today, writing, lecturing and learning while surrounded by his private forest preserve laden with healing plants.

If it's endorsed by Wood, it's worth my while to crack the pages and learn something about herbs and the Teasel Cure that Glidden alerts us to as the magic solution to chase those nasty spirochetes out from hiding. I have zero knowledge about the world of tinctures and natural pharmacopoeia, and this book just arrived yesterday. I'll pick up my own writing after I finish Storl's book, probably in a few days.

A German-based Teasel Elixir has arrived by La Poste

mail this morning, so with those other nutritional support formulas on their way via Billings, I should be all set to begin the complete program and get the show on the road by early next week.

I'll be back before then to report to you on Storl's writings.

Teasel Root Extract or Teasel Leaf Tea. Who would've ever thought? "Weeds In the Ditch".

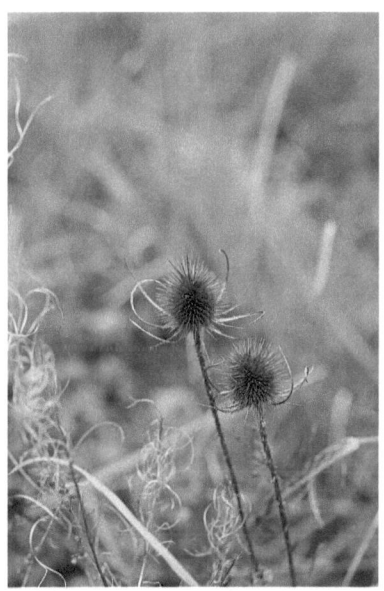 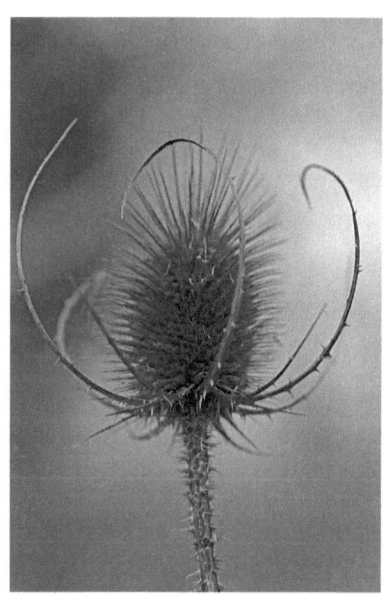

Wild Teasel, December 01, 2015
Found growing in a roadside ditch less than 250 meters from our home, and James Redfield's message strikes again.

Saturday, December 05, 2015, p.m.
11 days until my Périgueux Surgeon's Appointment

Much to report back to you since beginning Storl's book.

It's 349 pages cover to cover and I'm only on page 109. It's not because I'm a slow reader, but partially because of massive fatigue that sets in early each afternoon. After I let out the dog, get our daily fire nicely set, and a morning bite to eat, I continue editing the previous pages and then continue reading Storl. By mid Afternoon by brain is spent. At best, I get in a full hour's reading each day. But to be fair to my compromised brainpower, Wolf's book is a packed showstopper not to be rushed. Each sentence, each paragraph needs to be fully simmered and stirred in the brain pot to extract his wisdom. It's not a light breezy book but it does read more like a mystery story than the scientific treasure trove .he has written. It's well referenced, and completely understandable by a non-science person like me.

Here's my short take on some of what I've studied and compiled to date on Lyme disease treatment with Teasel root: Lyme disease is the result of very nasty corkscrew-like bacteria called spirochetes, that once they get into the body, will burrow themselves deep into the cell structure and are virtually impossible to chase out or kill off after they dig into the tissue. They have near identical characteristics of syphilis: Nasty, debilitating long-term malaise that gets progressively worse and can eventually cause dementia and death.

The Teasel treatment essentially flushes these corkscrew creatures out of their deep hiding. Importantly though, it's further thought by scientists, that the Teasel itself doesn't actually kill off the bacteria. The Teasel is the soldier on the horse beating the bushes and flushes out these parasitic cowards in hiding. Moreover, it seems that antibiotics can't begin to get into that deep cellular level to touch them. They're the untouchables even if a person used antibiotics for months on end. Lyme bacteria are like cockroaches in the night: Hard to get at and tough to kill because we never get a chance to see them.

So what kills them off once they're flushed out by Teasel?

Our natural immune system unaided by any drug.

However . . . we need an extraordinarily strong system in place to knock these nasty bastards out cold once and for all. It's like we have to become an ultimate cage fighter to get rid of this Lyme disorder. That's where the nutritional protocol comes into play, preparing our immune system for the cage fight of its life: Lyme spirochete bacteria vs. Jim Lindl. That's the battle *royale* about to take place in my body. It's that simple for me . . . win or die trying and I'm getting ready to fight.

The Cartilage & Lyme Killing Protocol Begins

Friday, December 04, 2015
Day 1 On The Partial Cartilage & Lyme Combo Protocol
PARTIAL PROTOCOL:

EFA Fish Oil Capsules;
6 capsules; 3 times per day; total of 18 capsules per day.
Recommended Daily Dose:1 capsule; 3 times per day.

Gluco-Gel Caplets; (Glucosamine and Magnesium)
5 caplets; 3 times per day; total of 15 caplets per day.
Recommended Daily Dose:1 caplet; 4 times per day.

Tangy Tangerine 2.0;
(cage fighting food to kill off the Lyme spirochetes)
2 scoops; 2 times per day; total of 4 scoops per day.
Recommended Daily Dose: 2 scoops; 2.0 per day; per 100 pounds of body weight.

That's it for day one. No Teasel yet. More vitamins to add into the mix in days to come.

I'm 195 pounds so four scoops of the Tangy Tangerine 2.0 is right on the mark for suggested daily intake. This powder goes into a drink and has just about everything imaginable. Think of it like a mountaineer's multi-vitamin go-power juice. I like the fact that it has prebioitcs, probiotics, amino acids, trace minerals plus all the vitamins.

This looks to me like cage fighting food at its best, a good spirochete killer. Tomorrow I'll report more, because I can feel some stuff happening today. One day isn't a trend, two could be a coincidence, and three days is a ray of hope.

Saturday, December 05, 2015
Day 1 On The Teasel

I continued with the opening regime above, but also started the German Teasel Elixir. One tablespoon of Teasel mixed into eight ounces of water and consumed in four separate parts during the day. Two ounces of water and Teasel mixture each time. By late afternoon, the right knee, heat sensation was less than half . . . that's huge news, but here's the important mile marker for me today:

When I let out the dog for his evening pee, in pitch black, I shook my head back and forth to test for eye flashes. The visual sensation is like camera flashes popping, and at night, that motion will induce them 100% of the time and yet . . . nothing happened! Zero, nada, nothing! "Something's already going on in my body," I thought. I went to bed for the first time in months without lights popping in my peripheral vision, only thirty six hours after starting these products, 14 hours after drinking the Teasel.

I've had constant flashes since about June, 2015. They began about three years ago, but at first, just sporadically. Always in both eyes. About a year ago, they started occurring every day but not all day long. By June this year, when it was dark outside, they never went away. When I walked about in the house, my peripheral vision kept flashing like a constant camera strobe going off.

Here's my most recent blood work, from November 6, 2015, and it says there's nothing wrong with me. Nothing in the blood indicates anything but a very healthy balanced body and a trace of Lyme antibodies. I definitely know different. Like those critical signals in my mountaineering days, these signals today are screaming at me to do something . . . and I am. The Storl teasel and the nutritional protocol.

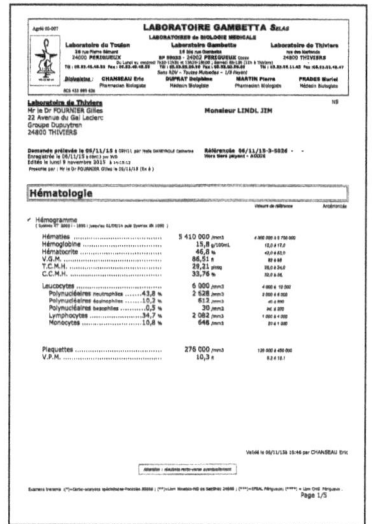 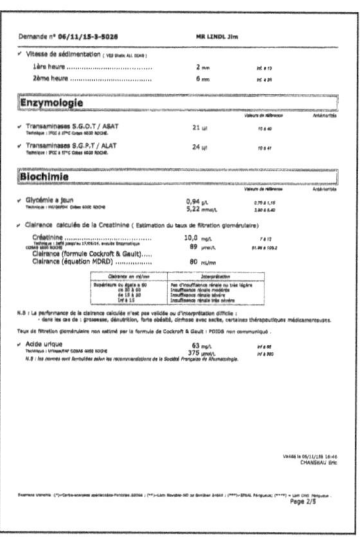

My Blood Work (p.01-02), November 06, 2015
© 2016 Jim Lindl

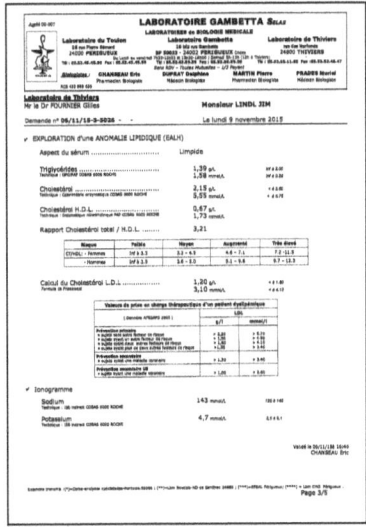
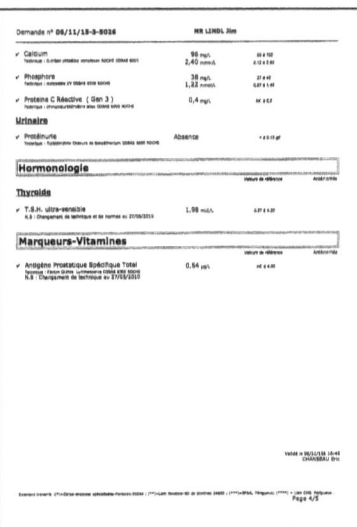

My Blood Work (p.03-04), November 06, 2015
© 2016 Jim Lindl

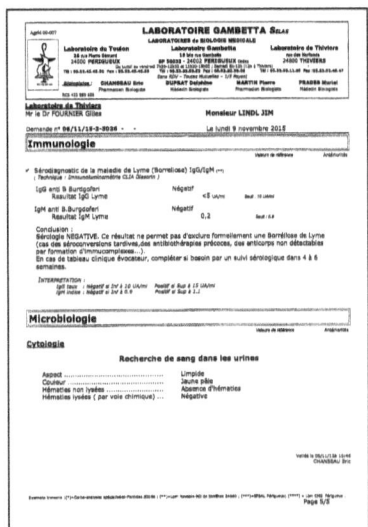

My Blood Work (p.05), November 06, 2015
© 2016 Jim Lindl

Chapter 5: Heavy Artillery

Here's what a month supply of nutritional heavy artillery and exotic European herbal phyto therapy looks like with an instruction manual how to win the war against Lyme disease by Dr. Wolf Dieter Storl, researcher and professor extraordinaire. Storl's book has become my lifeline and my bedtime Lyme healing bible. It's a must read. I'd be forever trapped in the Lyme dungeon without his experience and wisdom how to get out.

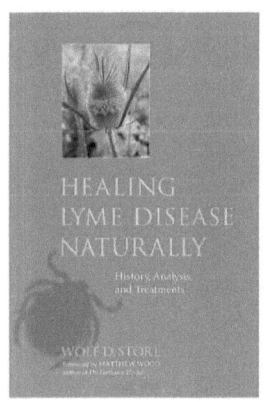

Healing Lyme Disease Naturally
History, Analysis and Treatments
by Dr. Wolf-Dieter Storl

Copyright © 2010 by Wolf D. Storl,
All Rights Reserved.

These following product images represent Herbal Phytotherapy and Highly Advanced Hi-Tech Nutritional Protocols of superior cage fighting food for both cartilage repair and the Lyme spirochete battle. It's a lot to swallow but thankfully it's all liquid or can be mixed into liquids and tastes pretty good.

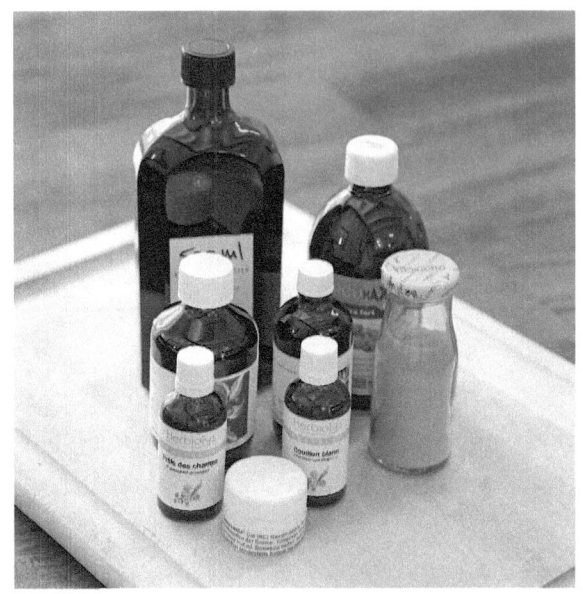

My Herbal Phytotherapy

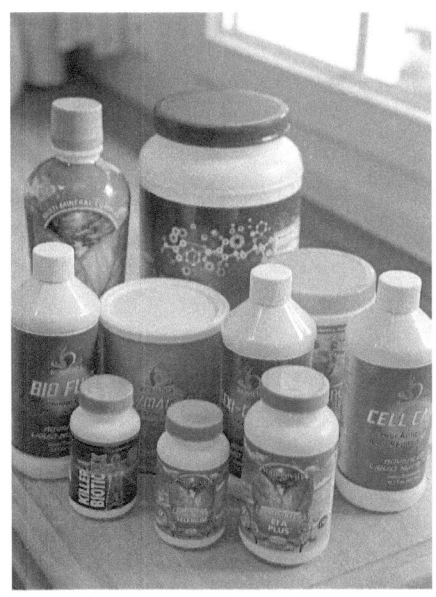

My Advanced Hi-Tech Nutrition

Our trip to California alone was 7,000 bucks to finally get properly diagnosed, without which I'd have no other alternatives except for a free hack and sew knee job here in France, but still with no solution for the Lyme maladies plaguing me.

The stem cell treatment is my back up knee option but it's not free and is a lot more money than trying some vitamins and an herbal concoction for a few months. Who knows. Moreover, at this point, I have no other options to alleviate my Lyme symptoms. Doctors in the States don't seem to have any definitive answers, nor do they here in France.

What with I've learned so far, I'd be crazy not to give this naturopathic route a good serious try for at least 3 or 4 months. The cost for airfares from France, rooms, food and rental cars in the States for a week is more than what these nutritional products will cost delivered right to our door here in France for the next 3 or 4 months. Plus, a stem cell job all by itself won't address Lyme bacteria, which I absolutely think are partially responsible for the rapid cartilage deterioration.

If I don't get those spirochetes and inflammation out of my knee joint, what's the medical logic of injecting more fresh stem cell food into the joint? Just feed these bastards another helping of freshly added cartilage? My plan is to smoke them out with Teasel weed and nutritionally kill them dead.

In that incredibly complex holistic process, my body can then begin to naturally re-grow cartilage back, one cell at a time. Some people say it's done all the time with this Teasel elixir and the high powered nutritional supplements sitting on our kitchen table. I'm about to find out. Yesterday, I've slowly begun to drink all these elixirs of Naturopathic promise.

I Can Feel This Stuff Working

Sunday, December 06, 2015
Day 3 On The Partial Cartilage & Lyme Combo Protocol
Day 2 On The Teasel
10 Days To The Périgueux Surgeon's Appointment

All of our bodies give off signals if we need more or should cut back on what we put into our mouth for life sustenance. Like water or booze… if too little of one, we get thirsty… if too much of the other, a hangover or a car wreck. The key is to pay attention to those signals before we heap ourselves into physical health trouble like I'm in now.

All of us have differing levels of perception and acuity of what's going on in our body because of a myriad of factors. Like a professional poker player or a hardened combat soldier, they probably have an acute ability to read their adversary because their life depends upon it. We're generally not finely tuned that way because our life doesn't depend on that level of acuity for much of anything these days. What goes on in our bodies is often a blur of perception that we pay little attention, unless we get ill.

If every day of our life, like ancient man, depended upon reading our body's signals, our tribe's signals and nature's signals to stay alive, we might be more cognizant to changes happening around us. I use to be that way for a period of my life. I offer up this side bar narrative to give you a feel for my expression "I can feel this stuff working" by day two. Let me explain.

I'll give you just two examples, among many, of extreme signal expression in the body I've witnessed or personally experienced myself.

Back in the day when I was enjoying a fairly high standard

of alpinism, the correct gear was important, the technical climbing know how was very important, weather reading ability was critically important, and physical conditioning a given, but it was knowing our bodies' individual failure nuances under stress that allowed us to get up and back down a mountain safely. For example in that picture of Mount Shasta, climbing from that encampment at Giddy-Giddy Gulch to the top takes about 15,000 calories and between eight and fifteen hours to summit and return back to high camp . . . given that everything works according to plan. It's pure human physics. March your body uphill 4,300 vertical feet, into headwinds at 40 mph, ambient air temperatures averaging camp to summit 8°F, and it takes a certain amount of energy to stay warm and accomplish that climb. At least 15,000 calories, and a certain amount of oxygen and water intake to burn up 2,000 calories of ready glycogen stores and another 5 pounds of pure body fat to create the metabolic process that fires the legs, lungs, heart and head for the round trip. On paper, it looks easy but in practice the hydration and fat calorie management to sustain that long steady burn rate, can be the single hardest challenge to get balanced just right given variable conditions, especially when a person is fifty years old.

When I was age 48, Zack, an acquaintance of mine from Wyoming, asked if I could guide him up Shasta in his 50th year of age, the following year. Although he had never done anything quite like this before I was game. He owns an underground utility construction company and has spent a literal lifetime in the trenches outdoors. He knows what punishing prairie winds and 20 below zero looked like days on end. He was fit and an avid elk hunter, never drank alcohol so I said OK, but read this book and report back to me every month with your progress, and we'll go next April, or May, snow pack dependent. The book was Mark Twight's *Extreme Alpinism*, the classic punishment regime of how to get in shape for serious world-class extreme alpinism. Mark Twight is a *Living Legend*, a man who personifies *Mental Kryptonite*. Mark Twight (Wikipedia)

I highly recommend reading some of Mark and let his mental toughness infuse your being whatever walks of life you travel. Mark to me is in the same rarefied league as Earnest Shackleton if he ever got into a major jam-up like Shackleton did in the South Polar Seas for 22 incredible months . . . and survived with his entire 27-man crew. Twight is in that type of league . . . super human, but also a leader extraordinaire.

In my day as a timber cutter, we were all tough as nails, really super tough mentally and physically, but not up to this guy's caliber. Not even close. Mark Twight is one of a kind. An ounce of Mark's mental kryptonite would be priceless if the pharmaceutical companies could patent the formula. It's all in the head Mark will tell you.

I wasn't going to climb with anybody unfit through avalanche conditions, and by June, Zack and I were ready, along with Steve, a third climber from New York State, who wanted back to the mountain for a second attempt. The first time Steve and I climbed Shasta together, conditions were unfavorable and we never summited but he came back for more, which is unusual for a non-climber, non-alpinist. I had him also committed to an 8-month pre-climb diet of Mark Twight. It showed. When he arrived at the mountain, Steve was a different person than one year earlier. Twight got into his head and he was now mentally tough, fit and ready to climb.

Most traditional alpine routes require an "Alpine Start" on

summit day. That's a climbing euphemism for rousting out of an arctic sleeping sack at midnight, getting roped up, into crampons, pack on and climbing with ice ax and headlamps by 1:00 a.m. at the latest.

Here's the point of all this preamble. When we climb at our physical limits, our body can break down and we stop. Failure is at the heart of pure alpinism. Alpinists all have to know their limits by experience. It can be deadly up there. This isn't a city jogging trail. No doctor, no scale, no electronic machine in the gym tells us where that limit exists. We learn this in the mountains. And limits are learned and exist because our water intake, stored fat energy, air density, all are metabolically mixed along with hundreds of other key elements like amino acids and minerals that keep our body firing up a mountain for fifteen straight hours with a 25-pound summit day pack strapped to our back all driven by ambition and desire. Each rigorous alpine climb is a lengthy personal experiment of sublime discovery.

On this particular trip of *sublime personal discovery*, we launched out of high camp and were swimming up the mountain in breezy textbook style all nice, slow, and safe. Shasta is notorious for heavy sustained winds and the ever-present potential for 1,000-foot icy death slides. This day didn't disappoint. That's why I like Shasta for training. It was blowing sustained 35 when we cleared Thumb Rock at 12,000 ft., and its intensity increased every step of the way up Misery Hill. By 13,500 ft. at the rounded airy apex of two steep apposing ridges that fall off either side into glaciers below, my Kestrel wind gauge clocked in at 72 mph. By then we weren't climbing but crawling in self-arrest with ice axes dug into the bulletproof ridge ice. Never before had I climbed in sustained killer winds like on that wind-ripped ridge with a 1,000-foot icy plunge below. Nobody was up high on the mountain that day. The lenticular told them to stay down.

But this was a special climb. Zack and Steve had trained hard for almost a year, traveled a long way and were very motivated to reach the top. I wasn't suicidal about it, but I pushed myself beyond anything I'd ever known before. The physical and mental drain and the intense responsibility for two rookies in those kinds of conditions is hard to imagine unless you've done something like that. . . It's not scary, not euphoric, but it can be surreal. I rank that trip as one of my most memorable climbs ever because of Zack. On the down climb, he and I, two grown men, teared up together. We survived by giving it our best. Mark Twight we weren't, but he would've approved of our grinding determination that day. His spirit was within us for sure.

It was at that moment at the top end of misery hill, 13,500 feet, climbing against 72 mph crosswinds, that my pipeline contractor teammate had his physical failure. He was smiling and could talk, he still knew my middle name, a standard test for dangerous hypoxia, but I could barely understand him in the roar of the wind. A huge lenticular cloud had formed on the summit, which meant potentially higher winds ahead.

At this exact moment, we couldn't move up or down. Zack couldn't function on his feet. His legs wouldn't move underneath him. We were pinned. He tried water, he tried some rest and nothing worked. He had totally shut down. No going up or down at that point and we were in a dangerous weather situation eight miles from the parking lot, twenty miles from Shasta City with nobody on the mountain and no possibility of rescue in those hurricane wind conditions. We were ultimately on our own anyhow, as I believe we always are in the mountains, and in life.

We didn't have cell phones. The notion of a cell phone in the mountains, for me, disconnects the alpinist completely from his connection to the mountain and the climb. The pristine beauty, the pure clean esthetics of multi-day backcountry alpinism would be shattered by a ringing cell phone. It would be like making a call during High Mass in Saint Peter's Basilica. Impossible for me to even comprehend. We were in our own spiritual mountain church where conversations with God do occur, but not by cell phone.

With no other ideas, Steve offered up a small squeeze packet of a stacked carbohydrate product called GU and that's about what it tastes like. A Mark Twight staple. They're small, like a one serving tear pack of ketchup. Steve had one in his pocket and had learned about GU (GU Energy Gel) from *Extreme Alpinism*. I must have overlooked that page in Marks's invectives.

Here was a 50-year-old extremely fit and prepared man, totally immobile at 13,500 feet elevation that two people with a stretcher could never carry, hoping that 100 calories of GU was going to get him off that mountain.

The miracles of our bodies' complex functions never fail to amaze me. Zack squeezed that sticky cold GU into his mouth and like magic it lit up his neurons and somehow re-booted his entire system. In less than sixty seconds, he was climbing at full power. We summited, and then down-climbed to high camp, packed up and walked out to arrive at the trailhead by 10:00 p.m.

We had been climbing for almost 22 hours non-stop at that point to reach our van. 100 calories of stacked carbohydrate at just the right time in Zack's metabolic cycle, out of probably twenty thousand burned up that day by him, made all the difference for his body. Go figure. 100 calories of GU saved all of us. Little wonder it was an emotional day up high. We were happy that day. Zack turned fifty, climbed his mountain, and we lived to tell about it.

Another climbing trip on the east side of Mount Rainier was my turn to crash. It happened to me on the Emmons Glacier route on July 4th weekend, 1999, when I also climbed to failure. There was a huge lenticular forming over the summit as we topped out. Our technical outer shells were plastered with a beautiful white glaze of rime ice head to boots . . . we all looked like white ghosts. It was -5°F and blowing our frozen ropes horizontal at 45 mph plus and time to get down fast. Our team of 3 guides and 8 climbers, plus another 2-man team of Himalayan climbers, were the only ones to summit that day. The RMI guides were all shut down from coming up the Cleaver route on the other side.

Just as we down climbed the Emmons Bergschrund at about 12,500 feet, I ran out of gas. Total body failure like Zack experienced on Shasta. A full liter of water is all I needed to reboot and get down to safety. Sounds easy, but getting a single ounce of drinkable fluid at below zero temperatures in 40 mph winds on an exposed glacier when it's time to hustle isn't easy to organize with 10 other climbers all roped together and in full retreat. The take away from all this lengthy narrative?

Small things missing from our body can cause big troubles. Small additions to our body can also make big improvements. Small things in our body are vitally important. I know this firsthand. Essentially I'm just adding some very small amounts of vital nutrition into my body to make a big difference. I expect it to have powerful and significant results, like the GU or the liter of water, but in different mysterious ways that only my body will figure out. That to me is holistic natural healing, like we experienced up high in the mountains. I know this to be true.

A promotional link to RMI guides and some pictures of Emmons, plus their training guide and what to expect. Mount Rainier Programs (RMI)

I've never used RMI but I think they do a pretty good job overall. I started with AAI in Bellingham, WA, and stayed with them because they demanded a high standard of client self-awareness and client self-reliance in all their climbing programs. We hired these guides for their wisdom when to stop and keep us out of trouble beyond our capability . . . not to get us to the top.

On that Rainier Emmons climb, an intrepid 26-year-old young man was lead guide. He was a seasoned Alaska Range guide who gained major experience from a very early age and then from hundreds of other guided summits worldwide. He reminded me of myself when I was a young timber cutter, experienced far beyond his years. Today he's gone on to become a private contract jet pilot and aviation broker who does extreme endurance off piste adventure competition in his spare time. I remember him and that climb well because of my systemic body failure up high. He made sure we all got down alive. I look upon all these gifted holistic healers individually, as that kind of rare guide . . . lifesaving guidance through their deep level of actual experience. American Alpine Institute

That type of mountaineering used to be a central part of my life. It's the reason I got seriously in touch at a much higher level with my body chemistry. Like racecar driving finds the limits of a car's mechanical ability, mountaineering will test anybody who pushes themselves to the max.

With that level of physiological system acuity developed

in the mountains, I can now usually feel very subtle body changes as they're happening. With this passage as referential back-story, I'll report my health progress to you as I perceive them occurring during any changes that I think are present . . . big or small, profound or trivial.

Monday, December 07, 2015
Day 4 On The Partial Cartilage & Lyme Combo Protocol
Day 3 On The Teasel

I've had no negative response in two days to all this heavy nutritional input, so today I added in the rest of the full Protocol. I wanted to give my body 48 hours to adapt to all this new supplemental influence. We're all different and I like to observe how my body is responding one step at a time. This is a heavy load of powerful nutrition for anybody to pour into their system all at once.

The Germans selling the Teasel have a suggested ramp up dosage on their Elixir spread over 8 weeks. It's probably pretty powerful stuff, which is good news to me. If I'm in a cage fight of my life with those Lyme spirochetes, I plan on kicking their miserable spiral shaped carcasses right out the door through my pee stream once and for all.

A Flash of Hope

Monday, December 07, 2015
Day 1 On The Full Cartilage & Lyme Combo Protocol
Day 3 On The Teasel

I began what I call the Healing Protocol, which is a heavy artillery barrage of everything but the kitchen sink as far as nutritional supplements. I'll list them all out later. I know it's heavy because through my distribution enterprise I started 24 years ago, I sold far more than a hundred million dollars of my vitamins back in day. In today's inflated dollars, that's at least a quarter of a billion dollars down Americans' throats. Among all those customers, tens upon tens of thousands of Americans, I never heard, thought, or suggested that a person needed such a heavy blast of nutritional firepower that I'm about to experience myself. But then again, I never helped anybody kill off Lyme disease or grow knee cartilage back to normal. Plus, I didn't know anything about herbal therapy. So, Dear Reader, it's a brave new world for me too.

Over the course of this journey, you'll get a good feel of all the different symptoms that have cropped up and I'm dealing with, but for now let's focus on these two: "Lightning like" behind the eyeball, flashes, and a constantly hot, burning sensation that surrounds my right knee. For the past month, my left knee is starting to heat up as well. So here's what we're watching for now. Constant Lightning flashes in both eyes and one hot, right knee

FULL CARTILAGE & LYME COMBO PROTOCOL:

Tangy Tangerine Powder 2.0
4 scoops per day; mixed with water; spread over the day;
1 scoop per 50 pounds of body weight.

Gluco-Gel Liquid
4 ounces per day; mixed with water; spread over the day;
1 ounce per 50 pounds of body weight.

Gluco-Gel Caplets
15 caplets per day; spread over the day.

Beyond Osteo FX Liquid
4 ounces per day; mixed with water; spread over the day;
1 ounce per 50 pounds of body weight.

EFA Fish Oil Capsules

6 capsules per day;
3 capsules per 100 pounds of body weight.

Liquid Plant Derived Minerals
2 ounces per day; mixed with water;
1 ounce per 100 pounds of body weight.

Killer Biotic FX Caplets
4 caplets per day; 2 times per day;
2 caplets per 100 pounds of body weight.

Selenium Caplets
12 caplets per day; 2 times per day;
3 caplets per 100 pounds of body weight.

HGH Youth Complex
2 bottles per month.

Z-Radical
2 ounces per day; mixed with water.

Alcohol-Based Teasel Root Extract,
As per label instructions & Storl's recommendations;
Daily for 2 to 3 months.

No doubt, this looks like an enormous amount of different products to the uninitiated to Holistic healing. But remember, I'm dealing with 2 things simultaneously. I have Lyme disease symptoms, very nasty and difficult bacteria that antibiotics can't touch plus cartilage repair. I'm going for the double header with heavy artillery.

If you go back and review the first video lecture on joint disorders, you'll find a less extensive list for just the cartilage re-growth and joint repair.

I'll report back tomorrow if anything of importance occurs. In the meantime, I'll continue reading Storl on Teasel and Lyme.

Tuesday, December 08, 2015
Day 2 On The Full Cartilage & Lyme Combo Protocol
Day 4 On The Teasel

I continue the full load as specified above. Throughout the day, I simply mix everything together in mountain spring water and down it. Mostly the entire concoction tastes pretty good, maybe a bit herbal for the uninitiated. The fish oil pills are another story. I never in my entire life could swallow pills . . . panic gag reflex . . . so I chew them whole. Pretty nasty until I got past the first 30 in two days. I just have to remember my logging days, my mountaineering discipline and this simple mantra: *This is easy because I can do it . . . this is easy because I can do it. Hard is when I can't do it. Be thankful for easy.*

It's In The Vibrations

I do drink the Teasel separately for a reason and here it is:
My belief and partial understanding how a lot of stuff works is predicated upon the inherent nature of energy frequency or vibratory cycles present everywhere: Far beyond our own Galaxy of stars or below even the deepest atomic shells and their densely packed nucleus . . . lies a hidden world of vibrations and energy in motion. Everything in this universe has a defined vibratory nature: Think about the basic interlaced energetic bond between 2 hydrogen atoms and one oxygen atom that forms a water molecule, think about the frequency wavelength of a microwave field of energy exciting a water molecule into a boil state in our kitchen's microwave oven, think about a frequency that a cricket or a dog can hear but we humans can't, or think about a cesium atomic clock used to time multiple GPS triangulation signals pinging from an iPhone to satellites and back to earth at the speed of light

to give us instant real time moving position. Incredible, all of it. It's all in the calibration, the measurements, the reception and the unseen interaction of these vibrations deep within atomic structure that lie unknowable mysteries resident in their sub- atomic whirl. Atomic Clock (Wikipedia)

We have four known energetic forces, power forces in the universe, that anchors all of modern science together and we haven't begun to understand the origins of any of them . . . *Magnetism, Gravity,* the *Weak Nuclear Force,* and the *Strong Nuclear Force.* That's it. That's what running the entire show for the last 15 billion years across the entire universe and we don't have a clue where these prime forces originate, or what powers them. We very well know *what* they do, but don't know *how* they get their power to do it. What keeps magnetism or gravity going from the origin of the universe to beyond eternity, or subatomic structure whirling and ticking like kryptonite glue from the bottom of the Grand Canyon to the edge of our Galaxy and beyond throughout the entire universe . . . is pure mystery and speculation to modern scientists. These forces "just are", according to scientists. For the most part, work-a–day mortgage payment to mortgage payment industrial scientists call the origin of these forces unimportant, irrelevant or they just avoid any thought of these deeper mysteries. Personally, I think about them all the time. To me it's a very big deal and central to forming core philosophies about a lot of stuff to try and understand where these forces of the universe began or came from or how long they may last.

The mystics and shamans, the soothsayers and other sundry prophets tell us it's all elementary. These incense burners have it all figured out and that certitude draws abject ridicule from the smart ones who burned up their family inheritance plowing through eight years of advanced enlightenment called a PhD in science. This academic crowd says science will eventually figure it all out, while the other group wearing togas claim there's a *fifth* force that powers the whole shebang. They call it God, or spirit or something pretty nifty that's pulling all the strings. For the past several hundred years one group walks off the stage with the prom queen, gets all the university grants, fancy titles, community status and Nobel prizes for attempting to identify some basics as to the origin of these four primal forces. They haven't even come close, yet they've taken all the prizes nonetheless. When some of these theoretical luminaries got near the end of their chalkboard life, they had to eat some humble pie and admit that maybe the incense burners had it right after all because these very same scientists didn't get a smidgen closer to finding the source of these four basic forces that power the entire universe.

These folks in togas and sandals usually don't even get an honorable mention from the scientific judges. These high priests of atheistic-based science mostly denigrate the crowd with long bushy beards, who don't bathe often enough for their high intellectual standards and die rich compared to these silly philosophers. Little wonder they think they're not only clever, but are also justly rewarded. *There is a god* they say when the bursar squeaks in another quarterly installment for more research, even if they don't believe in the deity they just blasphemed, which is exactly my point: Everything we need in life is usually hiding in plain sight, providing we don't let our biases get the better of us.

Abraham Maslow, the noted contemporary psychologist covers the reasons behind this conflicted dichotomy pretty well and in fact, I just revisited Maslow's writing last week for a booster shot of his thinking in *Religions, Values, and Peak-Experiences*. It's heavy reading for even Maslow acolytes. As an example, the 1st sentence on page 87 of this essay clocks in at 108 words. That must be a near world literary record. Most of his stream of consciousness writing runs 50 to 80 words per sentence. Not easy for me to follow. I'll bet he lectured that way in class too. Not exactly Socratic. I respect him even if he's tough to follow.

Maslow, to me, correctly articulates reasons behind this intellectual chasm between the 2 camps, i.e., the spiritual and the scientific. Like a tennis referee from his respected high academic perch Maslow beautifully finesses out the reasons for the now centuries old rift between those seeking truthful discovery. Storl in his Teasel book also has a few thoughts about the matter as well . . . He says the Teasel's secret might be in its vibrations which makes total sense to me because he has a bushy beard. I'm in his camp and trying to learn more from him, but the ultimate proof is in the spirochete death pudding for me. Abraham Maslow (Wikipedia)

Back To The Teasel Shots In The Morning.

My gut feeling is that if this micro bit of herbal Teasel essence has to go down the hatch for a cage fight with the spirochetes, I don't want to get it simultaneously confused or sidetracked with the myriad of nutritional frequencies radiating off the nutritional heavy artillery. I take the daily first shot of Teasel Elixir separate on a completely fasted stomach, about an hour before anything else. I drink it out of a pure silver challis in respect of whoever is pulling the strings out in the universe. I have to give somebody some sort of credit for putting that plant into my life. Why not credit first billing to the string puller?

Hey . . . why can't I lift a silver challis in reverence at my little private ritual? You think I'm not qualified? I believe in private ritual, moreover, I further believe it's not at all necessary to pay a high priced holy guru in some 1,000-year-old cathedral to sanctify my intentions for bodily healing. I have my own little Teasel ritual which I like and believe helps the healing process.

So I treat the Teasel tincture like a nitroglycerin pill placed under the tongue for immediate delivery. I want that Teasel to travel the most direct path to the fight arena, uninhibited wherever it has to do battle. I figure by swishing 2 ounces in my mouth, like an early morning mouthwash, for a minute or two, gives it a good opportunity to absorb nicely under the tongue and get to work immediately. No stomach mixing and degradation or intestinal delays or dilutions. That's my theory for taking it separately before anything else. But who knows.

The bottom line for me: I don't care how it works and 10 newly minted PhDs will probably never figure it all out from a "scientific" point of view anyway. I just want results, like Storl suggests is in the cards. I want to get rid of my Lyme bacteria and I'm trusting my body and the spirit forces of the Teasel to get to work pronto.

Here's what I have to report as of 10 a.m., December, 8, 2015 a little over 72 hours since beginning.

No hot knee syndrome. It's gone. That's 2 full days without a hot knee. The bone on bone contact sure didn't go away and it still has a grinding pain when I walk, but not the intense hot feeling. The heat is totally gone.

The eye flashes . . . none last night when I let out the dog into the dark of night for his evening pee. I've had these flashes intermittently for over a year and constantly for the past many months.

This morning as I swung my legs out of bed I immediately shook my head side to side to try inducing some flashes. I got a couple of tiny flickers on the periphery of both eyes. That makes two full days in a row with 99% of the intense eye-flash lightning now gone. "One day is a happenstance, two is a coincidence and three is a ray of hope." Tomorrow will be the third day. That Teasel must be down in the cage doing its vibratory battle with the spirochetes. Literally, rattling their cage.

Time for reading more of Dr. Wolf Storl and also tuning into the extensive webinar archives at the site here. Glidden Healthcare Advocate Info

This Naturopath has numerous, full one hour long archived webinars and podcasts of different maladies A to Z., and with winter in front of me, and nowhere to go but this chair and computer screen, I've got plenty of material to review since I'm now retired here in France. More updates later today or tomorrow morning. I signed up for his $20 per month subscription service so I can read everything on demand 24/7.

I'm very encouraged after only 72 hours on these products. Very encouraged indeed.

Tuesday, December 08, 2018, 2.24 p.m.

In the past two decades hanging around the nutritional world I must have heard or read the expression "colon cleanse" hundreds of times and yet I haven't a clue about how they work, what they do or how to do one. I can guess, but it all seemed too earthy to discover and more than I wanted to know.

I was never shy about outdoor squatting. We did it in those virgin forests at least once every single day, year round, rain or shine. Bears do it, why not us? Nature calls. My plumbing always seemed to function just fine. After finishing this passage, I'll have to link over to Glidden's site again and see what he has to say. I'm sure he has a webinar on colon cleansing.

Anyway, back in February of 1972 while hitchhiking back up from Mazatlán, Mexico, after being on the road for a month, I accepted a hit off a joint from the truck driver who was giving me a ride north back up to Montana. That was a different era and yes, we did inhale. It was a mistake. It must've been laced with speed or something pretty wicked because I had a most effective roadside colon cleanse in the snow as soon as I got dropped off by the Boise airport turnoff in full view of Interstate Highway traffic. It was a while before I caught my next ride . . . About ten hours later . . . after babbling at the passing traffic all day. That was the first and last "cleanse" until five minutes ago . . . and it was the equivalent of the Boise blowout. I'm not sure how or where all those spirochetes are going to exit, but I'll leave all the doors open if they feel it's time to skedaddle.

Tuesday, December 08, 2018, 5.24 p.m.

Been feeling better today than in a long time and it was time for the evening dog break when I unconsciously struck off across our level grassy fields for the dog's 2nd daily poop outing. Walking Stick in hand, I walked one fence line to the top, traversed to the opposite side and followed the fence back home, about 500 yards in total. It was a big mistake. My knee isn't hot, but the right knee pain is worse than it's ever been. It's killing me again. Instead of using my wheel chair for the dog walk, I simply forgot how bad that knee has been and just took off walking. It's as bad as ever. Maybe the heat is going out but it has a long way to go to be considered usable again. Now I know my benchmark of improvement. If I can walk that 500-yard circuit, without pain, something is definitely improving in the knee joint. That walk will be my gauge to indicate any new cartilage rebuilding. All I ask for is 500 yards across a grassy meadow with no pain and I'm home free.

This all occurred about 80 hours after beginning the nutritional healing protocol, including the Teasel four times per day as per the instructions on the German bottle.

Chapter 6:
Teasel Lightning

Wednesday, December 09, 2015, 3:30 a.m.
Day 3 On The Full Cartilage & Lyme Combo Protocol
Day 5 On The Teasel

I woke up early and slipped downstairs to put a couple of logs on the fire to hold it until daybreak.

Started the 1st of the 4 Teasel shots early today. By itself again. I like that segregation routine . . . Back to bed for a few more hours and will commence with all the heavy artillery later.

Last night I sent Dr. Storl an e-mail through his website. I feel the need to contact him. Without being too melodramatic, for those of you who have his book, please go to page 160, 3rd paragraph at the 2nd bolded line. On my 2nd day, I experienced the *lightning energy arrows* identical to what he described happened to himself . . . Exactly like his experience!

What's interesting and experimentally validating for me, is that last Saturday when the energy lightning happened, I had read no further than fifty pages in his book and had no prior knowledge of his thoughts on page 160 which I read late Tuesday, 4 days later.

When the lightning arrows shot out of my leg, I immediately commented to my wife what was going on. She was elated with the news, but not surprised, and said, "Okay!"

Then I showed her the passage about energy arrows in Storl's book. Incredible. She knows about these things. Her mother (from Eastern Europe) was raised in a culture of herbal healing and passed some of that philosophy down, mother to daughter. We've never practiced any of it, but my wife's aware how that type healing is supposed to work.

Very interesting . . . all of it.

Herbal therapy is definitely a new world for me to explore. If you're advancing through Storl's book and are fighting some biases, that's understandable. These herbs, I think, can be like fine wine: Hard for the uninitiated to understand what refined viticulture pleasure is until a person gets tipsy for the first time on a nice Saint-Émillion. Drink some Teasel if you have Lyme like me, and a person can begin to understand some of Storl's writing better. At least I can now. Up until a hundred years ago, the entire sweep of humanity used herbal therapy and sweat saunas as their centerpiece for health maintenance and disease control. They weren't naive, neither is Storl. Quite the contrary. Here is his website: Dr. Wolf-Dieter Storl - Cultural Anthropologist & Ethnobotanist

Wednesday, December 09, 2015, 12:39 p.m.

I'm on the second Teasel drink of the day and also fired off the second daily artillery barrage of advanced nutrition to get down to business, killing off those spirochetes. Teasel chases them out, the immune system kills them off, and out their carcasses get carted to the septic tank. A good proper place for those nasty bastards. Not to worry though, they'll all get recycled as food for the lawn via the septic drainage field by springtime.

Everything is good. No eye flashes this morning. None now, either. My breathing seems to be slightly deeper. I can definitely touch my toes much easier than five days ago. Remarkably easier . . . like down to the first knuckle touching the floor. Couldn't do that for years even with massive Egoscue stretching for the past 6 months. 5 days on this stuff and I can reach down lower a good four inches. That to me is remarkable. Must be muscle and ligaments loosening up nicely. Hasn't been that way for years.

My calf muscles must be elongating and loosening up with all these vitamin potions and elixirs. It feels important and good to reach deeply down to the earth level and connect for one or two seconds.

Massive Fatigue, Fuzzy Brain, Low Motivation

Wednesday, December 09, 2015, 4:24 p.m.

I just came in from outside . . . a nice sunny day. Storl suggests that besides sleep, calm rest, fresh air and all the other critical imputes of convalescing a malady, one should get direct sunlight into the eyes. Probably a good idea in these dark December days especially since I've been living like a hermit mole since September reading and stewing behind this computer screen. So outside I went. But this next narrative is important. It's called story texture. It's a necessary explanation so you can understand and evaluate the degree of physical and mental changes that I'm going through as they occur. Let me explain:

In this healing journey, I could make a statement like, "I'm thinking more clearly today." Well I can't weigh clear thinking on a scale and show you the results. Heck, I could say that to my wife and she'd likely have no idea to what degree or exactly what that means unless I put a reference beside it as a measure that she or anybody could understand. For example, if I told you that, "I know I can think better, because today I did a crossword puzzle for the first time in two years," . . . now you'd have a reference to timing and relative gain in my clearer thinking or diminishment of fuzzy thinking.

If a month from now I reported that, "things had really gotten better in my brain," you'd again have no reference, but if I tell you I'm now directing a development team of ten genius Russian puzzle masters on the Internet to create new and exciting crossword puzzles, you'd either think I'm lying or you have at least a relative understand of something that's otherwise pretty nebulous, "I'm thinking much better than a month ago."

In the future, I'll always try to add decorative back-story as texture so you can better weight my progress reports today and for the months to come.

Here is what I noticed today: My brain's definitely not as foggy as it has been for months and my motivation level is beginning to come back to normal levels, unknown to me for many months. Let me explain:

I got on the lawn tractor (my twin cylinder gas powered wheel chair) and worked on our grounds for two continuous hours today of grass cutting. I felt motivated, focused and happy. I could easily twist my torso in the tractor seat at the end of each dump cycle to reef on the lever that empties the grass catcher into the compost piles. This is very significant because we began hiring a service to do all that work since June. This afternoon I was focused on efficiently working systematic cutting patterns through the orchard, around the gardens and the grapevines, around the trees and flowerbeds, up the hill to the mailbox. It's all quite convoluted with three separate compost piles and a myriad of sectors to cut. It's a thinking exercise, not just a mindless back and forth routine effort, like cutting a flat municipal soccer field. This complex yard with side slopes, fences and landscape features takes conscious effort to cut safely and cleanly. I did all that today in professional like accuracy after being on these products for only five days. Remarkable I thought. I was happy today for the first time in months.

Last June I had to give up grass cutting because I just wandered around the yard on that tractor in a fuzzy stupor. My wife took over for whatever parts she could cut. I knew I was in trouble but didn't know why. We hired somebody to take over the yard maintenance.

One of the big tells of Lyme infection is massive fatigue, general lethargy and mental fog. Not just getting tired, but unusual deep chronic fatigue. Up until this September when I found out I had the Lyme malady and began researching it fully, I thought I was just getting old fast. In fact, that's the first thing I told my California Doctor when he asked me how I felt. I said, "David, I feel old." He said, "You're not old at all." I responded, "Maybe not, but I feel like I'm old and broken down." This was mid-September, 2015. I knew I'd been sliding progressively deeper into this pit of fatigue little by little for years. It was obvious to me because I was doing less and less physical work month by month. It had become a fight to do the most basic chores like take the recycle bags up to the community dump bins. Or things like cutting the grass, or rototilling the garden. I had lost my motivation to do those essential activities that I always enjoyed. I just didn't have the energy to do these simple things anymore. I blamed it all on my sore knee.

I could also see my deteriorating condition in comparison to how all my farmer neighbors worked, many older than me.

One farm owner who has rolling forestland and cow pasture right across the stream from us was reworking his barbed wire fence line in October. I know him very well. He helped us install a full kilometer of our own new fence eight years ago when we bought this place. I know what it takes to build fences because I've done it with him. Eight years ago, he and I cleared the entire property boundary lines of brush and brambles, installed 490 wooden pointed posts, 4 access gates, and strung 2 top strands of barbed wire and continuous woven sheep grillage around our entire place. I was 55 years old and my neighbor was 59 at the time. That was December, 2007, eight years ago. Today, I couldn't begin to pound in a single post or reef a strand of barbed wire taught and staple it to the post. Not in a million years.

Yet, just a few weeks ago I watched him performing, on his own property, exactly what we had done eight years before. He was energetic, focused, and worked steady on repairing his fence line. He's three years older than me, and I watched him work on an overcast fall day reefing on strands of barbed wire and pounding in chestnut split rail posts into hard ground. It was about five in the afternoon when he finished up for the day. I watched him across the river from my rocking chair on our porch with my birch walking stick beside me for assistance. He asked me how I was doing these days, I told him I found out I had *la maladie de Lyme*. He nodded. It's common in this area. He told me that a friend of his has had it for years and he's always *fatigué*. He then asked if I had a local doctor. I told him who and he said he's one of the best. I'm 63 years old and I felt broken and used up like my life was coming to an end as I watched him effortlessly put his heavy tools and rolls of wire back into the truck and drive off.

I don't feel that way today, 2 months later, after taking these products for the last 5 days. Cutting grass was a good day today. It too is now one of my new benchmarks of recovery. I'd be quite happy if I can continue cutting grass. Time will tell. Unusual weather this fall. In the previous 7 seasons, grass cutting always ended mid-October. Never later.

I'm Getting Excited!!!

Thursday 10 December, 2015, 2:40 a.m.
Day 4 On The Full Cartilage & Lyme Combo Protocol
Day 6 On The Teasel

Check out this link about Fish oil and why it cuts down pain and inflammation and is very beneficial for helping re-grow cartilage. It's from the Stem Cell clinic in Denver, Regenexx, referenced earlier. These guys are on the ball with their timely and effective Internet communication platform. I can definitely learn from them how to broadcast a message over the Internet. Maybe one day they'll read this journal and want to comment. How Much Fish Oil Should You Take for Your Arthritis and Stem Cells? (Regenexx)

After reading this explanation by these MDs about taking higher doses of fish oil pills, I can better understand why there's a fish oil component in this knee repair protocol. It's critical for overall good health. In all my years as a fully engaged vitamin executive, I never took essential fatty acids in my supplemental diet. Never once. How ignorant is that? Pretty ignorant!

I thought the nutritional protocol was a bit excessive in its specified dosage, but these Denver specialists who are doing stem cell repairs now have 22,000 patients that have gone through their different clinics utilizing their specific treatments since 2005. That's a lot of folks to observe post treatment. These docs in Denver recommend taking even more EFAs than Glidden recommends and they explain it very well.

This fish oil I've been taking likely explains why my hot knee went away in the first two days of the protocol. These docs talk a lot about hot knees and what causes that condition. I'm getting excited that all this is coming together.

I'm signed up for this Denver clinic's free webinars and newsletter updates. That's how I got this info. They seem to be good educators and definitely stress the importance of nutritional support in re-growing stem cells before and after you leave their clinic. After all, their stem cell injection is about the size of a pea. That means, for eventual successful cartilage function to happen, we have to grow the rest. That's *exactly* what I'm doing as well.

However, I just skipped the expensive pea sized injection and the trains-planes side trip to Denver. *I'm relying* on what cells still remain in my knee to begin the re-growth process spontaneously. According to Dr. Wallach ND, no matter how bad a knee is ground down, there are usually always a few stem cells left in there to begin multiplying again . . . and they will, according to him. We just have to reboot the growth process, with big doses of specific nutrition, like fish oil and the rest of the suggested heavy duty nutritional regime.

All this EFA discussion might seem academic until something actually kicks in, like my hot knees getting better. For me, I like to know the "why" behind the results. This explanation seems to hit the nail on the head because my knees aren't burning up anymore.

I'm heading into to the kitchen now to down some more of those golden pearly beauties!!! And then, back to bed after

I stoke up the fire. Should hold until morning.

Thursday, December 10, 2015, 9:18 a.m.

I upped the dosage on the EFAs (fish oil pills) after re-reading the Regenexx analysis and discussion about the efficacious chemistry of fish oil on joint cartilage repair. I upped from six per day to twelve per day. Four gel caps three times per day.

Here is the site again on fish oil: **REALLY GOOD INFO.**
How Much Fish Oil Should You Take for Your Arthritis and Stem Cells? (Regenexx)

My wife is going to wonder what got into me last night at 3:00 a.m. When I went to reload the fireplace, I realized the feed stack in the garage was down to a few bones of small wrist sized branches. Not big enough to hold a coal until morning. What to do? I got into the car, in the dead of night, and drove down to our main multi-year pile of dried firewood beside the garden area, pulled back the cover tarp, and loaded the back of the Scenic under headlight. It's a crossover hatchback Renault and a great vehicle. Probably the best one since I started driving a '52 Plymouth on the farm at age twelve. Yep, loaded it up, drove back to the house, charged the fireplace, and went to bed.

That's the kind of motivation I haven't had since I was a timber cutter on the west coast forty years go! Up at 3 a.m. stacking firewood in car headlights? Something is going on with my body and my brain big time! Absolutely 100%, this whole protocol of Teasel and nutritional heavy artillery has kicked in big time by day six. I hope it keeps working.

I'm Thankful

I think it's important to be sincerely thankful for all those things that surround us or come into our path of life that allow us to live a good, and balanced, and happy full life. I wasn't thankful that way when I was younger. I had to learn some lessons first . . . and I did from a Vietnam Vet fresh back from combat in September, 1971, in Kalispell, Montana.

Storl writes about this too. He thinks we get better or fuller effect of all herbal remedies if we stop and say some nice things or think some nice thoughts about the how and the why of this whirl and mystery of healing that's a gift of nature to us all. I never use to believe any of that stuff was important. In fact never even gave it a thought that being thankful was important until I roomed for a few months with that Vietnam Vet. Work hard and pay your taxes . . . that was my early success formula in life. I didn't know what thankfulness and gratitude looked like. I was too busy fighting through life chopping down North America's last standing virgin forest.

I'll just call him Mr. Prospector, because that's what he is: A genuine climb-all-over-the-mountains rock hound and mineral finder. He's become a bit of a folk legend in Idaho, Montana, and British Columbia mining circles. This guy is one of a kind. The Discovery Channel wanted to do a feature special on his life, but he declined. Not his cup of tea. He lives in the mountains. He's not some story on a flat screen TV.

Well the Prospector and I got jungled up in a rental house for a few months in Kalispell that fall. We were winter roommates while I was taking a break from whacking trees on the Coast. It was great fun for both of us back then . . . Wildman Timber Faller meets Combat Vet.

I was 19. He was 26, a first lieutenant in the 101 Airborne fresh out of heavy Vietnam combat. He'd been to hell all right, but at that time, wasn't fully back. He had probably seen too much and needed some adjustment time to process back into his civilian life. He mentioned something about an early out and some decompression time in the Philippines to readjust. He said just one thing about Vietnam when we met: *"You don't ever want to go over there."*

That moment is an indelible imprint in my life . . . his haunting low voice I'll always remember. He sounded dark and ominous to me only that one single time. I never heard that tone again. Never.

I knew enough from working with logging camps full of tough customers when not to press and to leave well enough alone. We talked very little about his Vietnam experience in those early days together. You'd never have known if anything at all was cooking inside him, because on his outside he quietly reintegrated while we roomed in a little three-room upstairs flat we called the Dog Farm. It was a memorable time for both of us. If you ever saw the TV series *MASH*, it wasn't unlike that, with the "Prospector" the star Dog. He definitely was the ringmaster and ran the circus to everybody's constant delight. He was beyond a friend, he was beyond a brother and he was beyond a mentor. He was a very special person who just showed up in my life by pure serendipitous coincidence while both standing in line where we struck up a casual conversation and decided to find a room to rent for the winter. That's how the prospector and I met.

It was from him that I learned what acts of kindness looked like. By his example, deeds, and conversation, instead of being angry at the world, he extended kindness like a red carpet for everyone to tread upon wherever he walked and whomever he touched. He touched me in those few months with his kindness and allowed me to see myself as a better person. He woke me up to become more considerate and be less self-centered. I was the angry one. I was the dark one seething with my own childhood toxicity and venom and I'm forever grateful to him for his influence upon me at the Dog Farm. I'm sure I'd have ricocheted through life from calamity to disaster if it wasn't for that brief time rooming together. We all need mentors at times in our life. He was there when I surely was in need. Serendipity struck once again while two strangers stood in a line together. What we need most is often hiding in plain sight . . . providing we keep our eyes peeled.

He turned 70-years-old just a few days ago and is also in need of new knees. They're shot just like mine, but he has two of them in need of a fix. We're friends to this day as close as we were 44 years ago. Maybe closer. His doctors say he's fully disabled by Agent Orange and has more stuff wracking his body than anyone would want to talk about, but yet, he's always thankful for every day of his life. The prospector is a person I wish I could be more like. He said to me once: It costs no more to be kind and considerate, and people tend to respond better. How true, but who lives that truth every day of their life? The prospector does. He'll be the first person to receive this completed journal, which I now know will be published someday. I can feel these products working, and it's only day six since I started.

I'm thankful to MR. TEASEL, Mr. Prospector, Dr. Glidden, Dr. Halverstadt, CK, and Dr. Storl. I'm grateful to all of humanity in this whirl of life to which we are in every way interconnected. Above all, I'm thankful for the mysteries of healing, wherever that source of power comes.

Chapter 7:
The Wait, The Healing

Time to take a rest from writing for a few days. Time to just let the Teasel and the nutritional artillery continue their deep cellular battle. I feel like everything is nicely in place for cartilage re-growth. Time for me to review all of Glidden's numerous archived webinars, and podcasts. He must have 50 of them. At an hour each, that'll take me up to and beyond my appointment in Périgueux with the surgeon next Wednesday, the 16th.

Dr. Storl's book is also calling to be further absorbed. I'm at page 170, the half way milestone on the road to his story's denouement. It's going to be a few days in peaceful retreat . . . a daily fire, food, and study . . . healing.

Study Material Completed During This Sojourn.

1) Dr. Glidden N.D. Knee Replacement Webinar. One hour in length. Covers all the basics of knee surgery and his holistic alternative, including his heavy artillery nutritional protocol plus much more. This is the very first tutorial for those faced with any concerns about joint pain or disorders. Mandatory viewing.

2) The second most, if not *the* most important webinar you'll ever watch for health and healing of Lyme disease. One hour long. He describes the entire artillery barrage to knock down Lyme bacteria. It's from this video lecture I was first

introduced to the idea of teasel root tinctures, and indirectly to Authors Wood and then Storl.

3) Dr. Glidden on Lyme disease.

4) Dr. Glidden on Detoxing the body of accumulated toxins
1) through 4) above: Glidden webinar library (by subscription only) Glidden Healthcare Advocate Info

5) Here is a recent article by Regenexx out of Denver. They're the MD directed powerhouse doing big stuff with stem cell therapy on knees. This primer on knee replacement surgery is very sobering and amplifies Dr. Glidden's concerns.
Knee Replacement Questions . . . (Regenexx)

6) More on painkillers, why my blood pressure shot up and the reason why I got off of them. Also from Regenexx.
American Heart Association Warns Of The Risks Of NSAID Use (Regenexx)

7) More on arthroscopic surgery and the inherent shortcomings of the procedure. From Regenexx again.
Knee Surgery Side Effects? (Regenexx)

8) These MDs definitely don't like Celebrex! From Regenexx again. They conclude that Glucosamine and Chondroitin are the proven answer. I agree. Dr. Glidden certainly does as well.
Chondroitin Better Than Celebrex in New Study! (Regenexx)

Some Thoughts On Storl's Book On Teasel

I've learned over a life time of various collaborative complex projects, such as my latest one with the iconic German Power tool Company, STIHL, that no one person has all the knowledge, abilities or the complete optimal solution of their own making. Life works best if we work together. Obvious in the extreme but often not practiced by the individual day to day. We humans can close our mental doors pretty quickly once we think we have it all figured out. I'm not even close to that stage with my current health struggles. In fact, I believe I'm just beginning, and ready to make course corrections on the fly as necessary. I'm paying attention to everybody I study, because my health state demands results now, not down the road.

Egoscue, the Paris marathon man, the prospector, my friend the Doctor guitar picker, herbalist Wood, friends in Montana, my wife, the company supplying the heavy duty nutritional protocol, the Teasel Elixir people in Germany, Regenexx in Denver, Halverstadt, Glidden, Storl . . . all amazing people, all with something important to contribute, combined with all the supporting cast to bring this story to this point is incredible. Incredible how things can work if we integrate in harmony and work together.

Dr. Wolf Storl is a must read, cover to cover for Lyme disease. The subscription based video webinar series, is also an important alternative naturopathic viewpoint.

The Regenexx information and articles are packed with good counterpoints to Orthopedic Surgery, in favor of stem cell treatment, and, as an adjunct to their technical treatments, they encourage intelligent nutritional supplementation.

Consider this e-book's resources to be like a huge banquet of intellectual food and nourishment that's best eaten slowly, chewed thoroughly, digested completely, from which complete absorption will occur, to the benefit of your transformative and new understanding that'll help you for the rest of your life. Chew, chew, chew . . . and then, chew some more.

Chapter 8:
My Green Mile

Tuesday, December 15, 2015, 3:37 a.m.
Day 9 On The Full Cartilage & Lyme Protocol
Day 11 On The Teasel
1 Day Before My Périgueux Surgeon's Appointment

I've been up for about a half hour, took a pee and put a fresh log onto the fire to hold until dawn. Pretty significant experience yesterday and it needs to be documented or the full texture of the experience will fade quickly. Back to bed for some more rest until daybreak.

It's 9:12 a.m. And I'm Back At The Keyboard

It was only 25 days ago I began writing this journal. Périgueux loomed larger than a steamroller in my mind back then. I'm thankful I've had the time and the wits and the wherewithal to retreat like this to find some truth that'll keep me out of the hospital.

I see the orthopedic surgeon tomorrow and I believe that day will be a mere foot note to this story because I can now clearly see hopeful daylight as I climb out of this grave. The casket isn't shut yet and the hole will need to be filled in . . . which I'm certain will happen as my strength and healing continues with all this vital life force flowing into my system.

This is Teasel Day 11 and I truly believe it has been engaged in battle with the spirochetes . . . big time.

Let me explain.

Yesterday at 3:00 p.m. I slipped out of the house with the pooch to catch some sun for few minutes. Storl says we need direct sun into our unprotected eyes to create vitamin D plus other energetic goodies that assist the healing process . . . so I usually sit out on a garden chair for a few minutes in the afternoon to reflect and soak up some healing energy each day. Sun time was the mission with my four-legged German buddy.

The upshot of that garden walk was a sublimely violent coughing spasm whose sounds ricocheted back and forth across our narrow valley. When I say sublime, think of *The Green Mile* movie scene with cell block guard *Paul Edgecomb* and the lovable spiritual death row prisoner *John Coffey*, who stole the audience's hearts, when he extricated that demonic energy field out of *Edgecomb* into his own mouth. Yes, Dear Reader, that's what it felt like yesterday in the middle of our grassy meadow on my way to the garden, but in a reverse flow outward from my entire body, not inward.

Witness to all this was our German Shepherd. When a person is a close companion to their third Shepherd dog in 35 years, that person knows the breed pretty well. Well even the pooch was mystified with my violent swings between retching and coughing. Well-trained Shepherds don't get riled unless they sense their own or the master's imminent danger. I can't tell you if our dog was concerned for himself or me because he kept his distance, which is unusual. He didn't have his tail between his legs, nothing like that, Shepherds aren't timid. They're fierce family protectors, at all cost. Hard to describe his reaction except to say he was very confused, as I was surprised at my *Green Mile* like eruptions.

The Bellowing Bull

I was bellowing a deep dry cough like nothing ever experienced before in my life. Not sloppy phlegm, not like food crumbs going down the wrong way, not a tickle at the top . . . this was deep and very dry and powerful. Like I had to expel something. Something wanted to come out but it wouldn't budge. Not up and out . . . it just wanted out through my chest. Like it had to burst out of the sternum and the solar plexus region. Not up through the throat but out of the chest through the fleecy shirt and the outer jacket I was wearing . . . like a Fukushima Reactor burst. I was expecting some sort of explosive force . . . but it never came.

I felt like that prisoner in *The Green Mile* wanting to expel *something* not meant to be in a human being. Something foreign needed to be pushed out. That was the coughing . . . Then the nauseating dry retching began. No fluid came up; just dry retching . . . even more decibels than the coughing. At first bent over and then erect, then bent over, and then erect again, and then bent over again. I bellowed like a bull moose in the woods . . . very loud and reverberating off the closed in valley hills that surround our field. I'm not sure I could yell that loud. It was like I was a wounded lion roaring at the whole world around me. No anger, no fear. No emotions at all. Then the second wave of coughing began like the first until it all stopped as quickly as it started. It was so sublimely violent it felt spiritual. None of this was painful. When this spasmodic fit ended, I actually smiled at the ridiculously unhealthy profile I must have presented in the moment. I was too convulsed to begin worrying about any of the reasons underpinning this spontaneous episode. The dog was more stunned than me and kept his distance until it all stopped. After it stopped, he wagged his tail and we were off like nothing had happened.

The whole episode lasted at most 90 seconds but it was spectacular, and it was just the beginning. The second act hadn't begun just yet.

The First Heat Treatment

Please understand this is Europe, and Old France to boot. We don't adhere to the obligatory daily shower regime that most North Americans' subscribe. Yes, I understand that culture. Back in the day, I probably did three a day. Morning, after a gym workout, maybe again before bed. Two per day for sure.

Here on the farm two per week in the winter is about normal. Of course, I *douche* the face and scrub up the hands and other parts as necessary, but Europeans consider daily bathing to be unhealthy. Who knows. I've slipped into this culture pretty easily and we do live longer over here than in America and have slimmer waistlines.

So for me to immediately *crave the need* to jump into the shower after that mid-afternoon spasm, borders on bizarre behavior around here.

Dr. Storl is a world-leading anthropologist first and foremost, before he added latter-day herb researcher and Lyme healer to his resume.

In his travels he's studied old European medicine back to the beginning of recorded ancient civilizations, and then further back into the prehistory Stone Age cultures, for their means and methods of killing off nasty stuff like syphilis, malaria and plagues, along with other sundry maladies of the day. Part of these cultures' near universal disease treatments, throughout the entire sweep of history, was the inducement of heat into the body by fire or heat inducing herbal concoctions, or both.

From Finish saunas and Russian steam baths, to native sweat lodges, to palm thatched steam huts in the Caribbean, they all seemed to be into heat treatments of some kind and for good reason. Back then, they didn't have Google to copy each other's ideas, yet different cultures still found their way to this common heat cure across oceans of time and distance with no communication among themselves down through the ages. Fascinating to me how good ideas got around very effectively long before the era of printed communication. Some of these very same ideas just seemed to pop up in different cultures without any means to access each other's knowledge base. Very distinct and isolated cultures often were using the very same healing methods that had no means of communicating across vast oceans of time and proximity.

According to Storl's research and hard clinical evidence, if the body is exposed to direct hot water contact or indirect steam temperatures of 107°F for a brief period of time, just about everything bad will get killed off. The trick is to survive the treatment by killing the bugs before a person gets a stroke and dies from overheating. I guess our elders rationalized that a person will *most probably* get killed by the disease bugs but *only possibly* be killed by the steam treatment . . . take your pick. It must have been with high probability in favor of the heat tent or the tribe would've done otherwise, just like big pharma pitching their drugs on TV.

Today, if too many folks go down with serious side effects from modern meds, big pharma backs off the TV pitch because the class action ambulance chasers will raid the company's cash drawer pretty quick and heavy.

The ancients were no different. If their treatments killed

too many in the tribe, they must have moved on to something more conducive to survival. Progress was made, but it appears they stuck with their steamy saunas and heat treatment ideas for the past 10 plus millennia right up to current time.

So I figured ten thousand years of "clinical study" called the human race survival can't be all bogus, so I took the 107-degree plunge in the shower until the boiler was drained. It was incredible how good it felt after all the retching and violent coughing out in the field.

The Spanish Royal court wasn't naive either. The French disease "syphilis" ran pretty high in those 16th-century Spanish circles of golden empire debauchery. According to Storl, at least 3,000 of these European Royals sailed on down to the Caribbean in their yachts of the day, specifically to take the heat cure for syphilis . . . and it worked reasonably well . . . it kept them healthy enough to keep that whole empire business running until they met their guillotine fate later in history.

None of this heat treatment thinking was present during my bull-bellowing and lion-roaring session out in the meadow. I just felt I had to scrub my skin clean. Get something off me. Scrape off a film of something crawling on the surface. I wasn't thinking Storl or Caribbean steam tents in the moment. I was focusing on walking the 200 meters back to the house and climbing into the shower to get clean.

Immediately into the shower I went, cranked it up as hot as I could tolerate, and stood there like a stoic leather mummy, water pelting down over my exterior and flushing off unseen toxins.

According to Storl, who I re-read after that shower, he says that Teasel works much better with some hydro heating swirled into the mix. He writes extensively about this type of worldwide therapy, including Vichy hot springs. So I guess underneath all that decadent pampering at the old French Nazi Headquarters some pure therapeutic treatment is going on after all.

After learning about the theoretical 107-degree hot water bacterial-killer benchmark temperature, I was curious exactly how hot the temperature was that I had locked into place on the shower knobs until I had completely drained out the boiler. Later, with a stainless steel Swiss digital chef's thermometer, I found it registered 107.6°F, sustained at the showerhead when run for three minutes or more.

I think James Redfield might be pleased that one of his long ago readers is taking his message to heart: Keep following all the breadcrumbs on the trail of life. They'll lead us somewhere good as long as we pay attention.

December 15, 2015, 5:49 p.m.

Tomorrow may get pretty involved after the Périgueux appointment. Not sure how it'll unfold, so better to get these additional keystrokes in now while still fresh in the mind.

The Second Heat Treatment

Back into the shower I went again at 6:00 p.m. for the second time today, and timed the directed hot water to my knee and head area. Storl talks about heating separate zones as opposed to plunging totally into the tub for a full body cook off. Safer from overheating the whole system.

This trip into the shower ran ten minutes total, split five minutes directly on the head with the rain bird at 107°F, and five with the pencil stream at 111°F directed circularly around the right infected knee. I took the meat thermometer into the shower with me to get accurate readings while the mummy got good and cooked.

There's a huge difference in heat strength perception with just 4 degrees of difference. The knee was cooked red as a lobster after five minutes at 111°F, and it felt absolutely cooked to the max. I know this is the right thing to do. It reminded me of the old logging days when the standard treatment for infection was to load a pan or tub with Epsom salts and keep the water as hot as could be tolerated until everything got good and wrinkled. Half hour was a common soak time. With that system, anything nasty just cleared up. I should have remembered all that when reading about heat treatments, but I didn't, until I was cooking that right knee today. It reminded me of those days in camp forty years ago. Very therapeutic feeling and the correct thing to do.

My theory of heating the head is twofold. First, we know from mountaineering that the head is a prolific heat exchanger because a lot of blood moves through the brain, second because of my eye flashes for the past two years, I suspect those spirochetes have crossed the blood brain barrier and are causing that lightning like sensation.

Neurological disorders are common when Lyme or Syphilis bacteria are resident. Hot Hydrotherapy may boost the Teasel efficacy according to research in the mater. I agree because of what happened thirty minutes later.

The Detox Begins

Detox is an interesting thing. When I'm done writing this passage, I'll hyperlink over to a video lecture site for some more naturopathic insight on the subject. This ability to crosscut back and forth off these pages is what I like about e-books format. If you want to get in depth about a subject, like detoxing, you can stop reading here, and navigate to somebody who knows what the heck they're talking about. I see Glidden has a webinar dedicated to detoxing. He must think it's pretty important if a whole webinar is dedicated to this one subject, and I agree. I've got experience with detoxing both on and off the job. Back in the day when I was fraternity liquor manager at the DKE in Edmonton, I learned a thing or two about detox. Most everybody does at least once if they went through university in the past 40 years.

When a person drinks a fifth of Southern Comfort too fast, they usually have a nice conversation with the porcelain telephone before bedtime. If we chow down at our favorite taco stand and heap on some questionable guacamole, again, a massive food poisoning can precipitate a headache first, then another conversation with the toilet. I believe those are episodes of basic toxin purges we know firsthand, or have at least heard about.

Storl advises us that, according to the research literature and abundant anecdotal evidence, a person on Teasel for Lyme bacteria will detoxify and sometimes quite violently. Here is a good place to link to if you have questions about detox. Glidden Healthcare Advocate Info

In this particular webinar, he does a fantastic job of educating us on the basic physiology of the liver, stomach, spleen, small and large intestine , and how they constantly interact to clean toxins out of our system.

I found out every drop of our heart pumped blood goes directly thought the liver. Later I learned from another source that the heart pumps 2 to 3 ounces per beat. In one minute, about 4 to 5 liters. In one day, 2,000 gallons! In 10 days, the human heart pumps the equivalent of a big sized swimming pool. Every drop goes through the liver. That's one heavy-duty 24/7 filtering system to get the whiskey, beer and GMO sludge all cleaned up and out of the building. Maybe it's also cleaning up the dismembered Lyme carcasses coursing through my plumbing works. Who knows.

He also talks about the function of rest and sleep in the repair process.

Finally he thoroughly outlines a sensible and easy to follow six day detox program that includes three days of food fasting. This lecture is an excellent primer. Highly recommended.

Storl covers it very extensively in his book and just like getting rid of Southern Comfort is a very good thing . . . so is expelling the toxic residue that occurs when the dead decaying spirochetes turn into a nasty flow of sludge.

Farting At Lake Helen

This day wouldn't be complete without reporting about my farting and mud pie episodes after the second shower today.

Most of my knowledge about farting has come from observing our dogs over the past 30 plus years and listening to lectures by the leaned physician who in his best-selling book claims to have advised Sylvester Stallone among other movie stars about proper diet, food allergies and colon health. He was the very same doctor who I traveled with cross-country preaching the gospel of our company's vitamins.

This is all earthy talk I know, but if you would've climbed with me on Shasta to Lake Helen, at 10,400 feet for the first overnight stop on the mountain, you would've known what real life humiliating earthiness is when you have to crap in full view of 500 fellow climbers, both men and women, then stoop down, scoop it up and put it all nicely back into your mountain pack, with all your food and clothing for the next four days. Helen Lake is just a name. There's no lake there. It's a stark snow-white plateau about the size of a football field behind a moraine bump where everybody camps overnight on this particular Shasta route, because of extreme avalanche and rock fall potential outside this very limited tenting zone. The route is called, "Avalanche Gulch" for good reason. There's not a rock, a tree, or a snowball to hide behind to do your business if you're up there for spring climbing. It's squat, drop your Johnson, poop and scoop, pack it up, put it away and get over it. Everybody does it in full view, in stark white brilliance against dazzling blue sky, for all to see.

Imagine yourself in front of a huge patio of sunning skiers at Squaw Valley, at the Lodge, having a beer and chatting on a nice sunny day. Then imagine yourself walking out in front of this crowd to relieve your brown and yellow urge. That's about what it feels like at Lake Helen. Same festive relaxing atmosphere, just slightly different behavior. I never did Woodstock or Burning Man, but their excuse is probably hallucinogenic drugs. These are sober church going climbers at Lake Helen.

If you're not quite up to this sort of humility, reconsider climbing up to that high camp launching zone on a weekend. Mountaineering requires deep motivation and is a test for a lot of stuff to get to the top. Pooper-scoopering after yourself like a dog in the park is the least of the obstacles in gaining the summit of Mount Shasta.

I recommend a few practice runs in the back yard before heading into the backcountry. The rangers will fine a climber and revoke their permit for non-compliance.

Here's a cute Ranger's tutorial if you can't broach the

pooper-scoopering subject with your friends who are organizing a climb up Shasta. Get used to this Rangers smiling face because you'll probably be meeting him up there on the mountain . . . crapping away just like everybody else in full view. The Mt. Shasta Human Waste Packout System . . . (YouTube)

According to this well respected and learned Doctor at the link below, who wrote a best-selling book about food allergies and colon disorders, smelly stools and farting are an obvious sign of less than optimal plumbing. Dr. Braly's Food Allergy & Nutrition Revolution (amazon.com)

Back in the early 1990's, when I was just awakening to the world of "alternative" health and healing philosophies, this book by Jim Braly really opened up my mind to this foreign holistic health world. Now remember I'd been on the road traveling with Jim while he kept our audiences at the edge of their chairs with his scintillating 2-hour lectures. This Medical Doctor was one of those rare gifted researchers and practitioners who could connect his clinical understanding with a lay audience better than anybody I've ever known . . . bar none.

He indelibly imprinted some of the key fundamentals that make us sick and the pathways to healing and staying healthy . . . and his truth has stuck with me ever since. If there's one book to read that'll hook a person, and begin to anchor their understanding and belief about eating correctly, this book is the top of my list. He's considered by many of his peers to have pioneered certain understanding, long before anybody else, the correlation between "leaky gut" syndrome, food allergies, and major health issues. If we don't get our digestive plumbing working properly, we are slowly dying. He has treated over 10,000 patients with what he writes about in the book. I'm one of them. Back to farting . . .

My German buddy usually turns and sniffs when he's done. He's checking his state of health. We need to do no less. Stool composition, color, smell, and deposit frequency on just a cursory visual level can reveal if something is cooking inside . . . so-to-speak. I suspect that astronauts have every drop of sweat, every heartbeat, every ounce of pee and poo analyzed in real time during their missions. Their life probably depends upon it.

Dog number one of ours used to fart so bad he occasionally set off the smoke alarms in our Sacramento House. Not a big deal except when the system is hard wired and can't be overridden at the switch box until the fire department comes or the methane dog gas is evacuated out of the hallway. He was a big dog. It happened a time or two.

So yes, I'm cognizant of changes in that type of bodily behavior, especially since I began this protocol, and I can report that things are "cooking" very unusually for the past two days.

Let me explain because it's very significant and I believe it's a sign I'm detoxing.

Yesterday, ten days into this protocol and the day before this Bull Bellowing episode began, I began to spontaneously fart a little. Toot, toot. That was it. But . . . a bit later, again. Then later . . . again. By the end of the day, both my wife and dog took notice. My wife because of the smell and the dog because of the noise. It became more remarkable as the day wore on . . . like the sound of heavy denim stitching getting ripped apart when a person dismounts off a tractor and their jeans get hung up on something and tear apart. That kind of unexpected serious, cloth ripping noise.

Now please understand my plumbing works very well

after Dr. Braly got my digestive plumbing all dialed in over 20 years ago. Ten little farts per year were probably about it until yesterday morning. Ten per year . . . Then yesterday, although not keeping specific count was probably gusting five per hour by dinner time and trending higher. By 10:00 p.m., when doing some Egoscue stretches, a major ripper cut loose that perked up the dog's ears. My wife heard it from the back of the house and remarked that it sounded like this old stone mill house was settling. Things were definitely cooking inside my guts.

Today was no different. When out in the field earlier during the bull-bellowing episode, the farts were in unison with the coughing and the heaving convulsions. It was wild, I tell you. Wild. No chunks, no liquid, no slime, just dry *staccatissimo* strings of farts. Yes, *staccatissimo* . . . almost *operatic!*

Into the shower I went. More of the same and continued up to the second shower. No chunks flying out, no nothing.

After the second shower the coughing returned, with not disruptive farts but definitely noticeable. About an hour after the second shower, it happened. A spectacular mud pie all dispensed nicely into the white porcelain ten-ring, neat and tidy. The Shasta Rangers would be proud of my superior accuracy. No muss, no fuss, no embarrassing over spray. The coughing stopped, the farting stopped and it felt like a lot more than poop came out. Who knows, but I'd call that a detox of some magnitude. I farted more in the last two days than the last twenty-two years since I did Braly's 30-day food allergy diet August of 1993.

Finally, after two days of farting, and dry coughing I had my *Green Mile* moment of purge. I knew right then who was winning the cage fight. Teasel became my hero. Mr. Teasel was kicking the crap out of my system, literally.

Editor's note: It was from this paragraph that this book's Title was born: *Mr. Teasel My Hero*. The original working title, *How I Dodged A Bullet*, was forever changed from this point forward.

"Something's working with this high powered nutritional protocol and the Teasel," I thought. The Lyme spirochetes were getting ambushed and were being carried off the battlefield in droves by every drainage system in my body.

Dear Reader, if you're having a hard time following this detailed narrative from the beginning of this chapter and are a bit repulsed at this juncture, I completely understand.

You haven't been pinned in a snow shelter for 48 hours up high in 100 mph hurricane winds with two burly fellow climbers like I have. This highly descriptive earthy behavior is exactly what goes on in a tent when three people are jammed into a space smaller than a queen-sized bed with no possibility to exit out into the storm to do our business because we would get blown sideways straight off the mountain. This type of resolute earthy banter in a storm shelter helps break down the fear in catastrophic mountain storm conditions. This is all part of a mountaineering experience.

Linked below are a few pictorial reasons why civilized normal office workers from San Francisco bust their butts and go through the punishment to climb Mount Shasta. Mount Shasta Avalanche Gulch (Outdoor Project) Imagine for a moment being on top of that mountain yourself . . . with some of your very closest friends for the very first time, sharing that sublime summit accomplishment together . . . it becomes easier to understand the powerful forces that mountains have upon climbing friends who scale the heights into the wilderness void of the pristine alpine world . . . to share something very pure, very spiritual together.

Chapter 9: Périgueux

Thursday, December 17, 2015, 7:52 a.m.
Day 11 On The Full Cartilage & Lyme Protocol
Day 13 On The Teasel
26 Days Since Beginning This Journal

The Surgeon's meeting yesterday was most excellent, but I'm not ready to write about it just yet. More time is necessary to fully digest what was discussed. Tomorrow I should be ready to put some thoughts into this journal. Better to sleep on it another day, because what I write here, will be my course of action going forward.

We live very close to the 45th Parallel North, which means it's dark outside and the days are short. We're four days from the winter solstice, the darkest day of the year, a special time and a good metaphor of my current station of life, the darkest time of my life . . . with re-birth an awakening of my healthier life straight ahead.

Some ancients taught that the Jewish Mystic of Nazareth was born on the Solstice. I like that idea. I'm Jewish by maternal birthright and share tangential lineage with him I suppose.

My strain of DNA, according to the National Geographic DNA genome project, says I'm of the ancient Ashkenazi Tribe of Jews that goes back 25,000 years into the Middle East. Makes perfect sense to me given what my mother told me near her death and later familial Internet research about her Tribe of people out of Trois-Rivières, Quebec. She emphatically revealed the biggest family secret never spoken to anybody, family members included, that her maiden name wasn't Greek after all. They were all Jews who changed religious affiliation at the behest of the Holy Roman Empire's not-so-subtle request in Southern France about 300 years ago to lose their Jewishness or face death.

That was called the Catholic Inquisition. At age 62, I definitively learned I'm a birthright Jew through and through and not a Catholic after all.

Who knows. My siblings might drop over learning that they've lived under a cloak of multi-century deception that large and for that long.

A lot of folks structure more than their spiritual belief around various religions. Just ask the Christians what they think about Muslims these days. Wouldn't it surprise some Christians if they had the courage to test their DNA with the National Geographic project and find out there are a few closet Muslims amongst themselves all along. Someday there'll be plenty in the closet if certain potential politicians get their way and chase them underground like my Jewish ancestors were by the Catholics in France during the inquisition.

The ancients certainly felt these periodic seasonal punctuations, as do our local subsistence farmers. I feel a transition happening in my life these past few days . . . but much more than a simple, pending change of daylight. It feels like my body, my mind and my spirit are passing through a wall that has been blocking me for a very long time. Maybe a lifetime or more. Storl talks about this kind of transformation stuff happening when a person drinks the Teasel to kill of the

Lyme. Who knows, maybe there's some sort deep spiritual battle taking place in my body. I'd be happy if I could just walk behind the lawnmower to cut the grass next summer

The Teasel Ritual

I've established a morning ritual with the Teasel that really feels good. Here's how it works:

First, I put a nice log into the fireplace to sustain comfortable ambient room temperature for the morning. After the firewood is nicely throwing off its stored energy collected from the sun decades ago, I wash my hands, water only. No soap.

The next step is to organize the vitamin arena and get prepared for the Teasel drink and Daily Nutritional Artillery Barrage.

The Teasel Elixir gets prepared with volcanic spring water, from Auvergne, near Puy de Dôme. Then the prepared mixture goes into a small silver challis and is ready for the healing ritual.

I sit in a chair up close to the fire with the doors swung wide open with penetrating radiant energy washing over my face, my body, my arms and legs . . . head to toe, but especially cognizant of the distinct power of the radiant energy wavelength penetrating my sore right knee.

A few minutes of deep settled rhythmic breathing follows which then initiates free passage into an unseen realm . . . known to all sincere believers. With the challis in both hands held between thumb, index, and middle fingers, a reverence is struck with the following silent invocation:

"May the divine Essence of the Cosmic infuse my being and cleanse my body, mind and spirit of all impurities, so that I may commune with

the universe of life, light and love, and all its wisdom and power . . . with the purpose of sharing your energy and gifts for the benefit of all humanity to live in harmony, but only if our intention is sincere . . . with great purpose and gratitude . . . for all thy gifts bestowed. So Mote It Be."

I drink the Teasel . . . and close the fireplace door to begin the day. It feels really good to have a nice little private moment without thinking about anything. Then the challis gets tucked back up into its silent little world with the other decorative china cups that keep it company.

After that little session of privacy, I then open up all the heavy wooden window shutters and let in the light of day to get on with the rest of my life.

Here's a pretty cool breathing technique, that's practiced by a battle scarred marine combat vet and helps him more than a daily hit of booze and happy pills, for his Gulf-War PTSD. Breathing: The Little Known Secret To Peace Of Mind, Psychology Today, April 14, 2013

Back To Earth For Another Day

If you're feeling a bit embarrassed or sorry for me by reading this passage above, don't be. My mental passport has traveled beyond the boundaries of River City and out into the wide world more than a few times. I'm very comfortable with whom I am because I know where my heart lies, and it isn't stuck on convenient superficial social pretense.

So here I am . . . back to earth again tapping this keyboard with a message of hope for somebody to read one day. I've begun to feel like I'm creating a multi-page directive pointing toward the *Lost Dutchman*, of truthful healing.

Yesterday in Périgueux was tremendously interesting and reassuring to me that I shouldn't go under the knife. I thank everybody in the universe that'll listen, for bringing me all this healing knowledge and Mr. Teasel to my doorstep. I'm thankful I had the wisdom to listen and act upon all these gifts that are changing my life.

The Surgeon's Meeting

Friday, December 18, 2015
Day 12 On The Full Cartilage & Lyme Protocol
Day 14 On The Teasel
2 Days After The Périgueux Surgeon's Meeting

The short version of what went down in the surgeons office: Met with the Doctor, a warm, affable personality that exuded confidence not arrogance. Fluent French, English multilingual speaker. Paris born and educated. Loves his work, loves his clinic and loves Périgueux.

This multi-disciplined 52-bed ultra-modern specialized clinic is attached to the regional hospital and is rated AAAA, (four A's), the top rating in France. This Clinic gets rave write ups because it attracts the very best doctors and has the post-surgery report card to back up its reputation. No question, I'm in very good hands here.

The Surgeon asked for my medical dossier, which included the current 2015 and earlier, 2008 x-rays plus all blood analysis, and a sealed general report from my local doctor who organized this appointment for me a month earlier.

The Surgeon looked over the two x-rays, talked about the difference in seven years, and said I'm at condition stage 4 and in need of reconstructive artificial implants: Cut here, and cut there, realign things back up, sew it all together, and out the door I go after a few days in their nice clinic with a fine view of the park. He had me walk around the room, then sit up on the table while he twisted and waggled both hips and knees. He said I'd be able to work on that knee after twelve months of rehab and recovery. "Twelve months?" I asked. "Twelve months," he repeated to both my wife and me.

Then It Got Worse

He asked for some detailed history on me. I left out everything about my current holistic protocol that I recently began, i.e., the Teasel, the Nutritional Protocol, the mud pies, the stem cell research, Regenexx in Denver, all the information that's linked into in these 147 pages over the past 27 days. I left it all out of our discussion for a good reason. I didn't want to challenge any of his thinking by offering up anything outside his comments. I was there to learn, not teach and preach. Over the years, I've found I can learn a lot more by acting naive than by showing off how smart I'm not. So I kept quiet about what I was recently learning through all the research talked about in this journal.

However, I did go into my Lyme symptoms chapter and verse that you've read about throughout these pages. That got his attention and the conversation shifted dramatically. He responded, to my thinking, like he was expertly triaging me in an MSF refugee camp in war ripped Afghanistan by his laser-focused decision making confidence. I'd bet you a hundred bucks this guy has done some MSF time in some hellhole some place. He seemed to have that spark of deep humanity for that type courageous compassionate work. I liked his personality a lot. So did my wife.

He said you can't have your new knee until we figure out what's going on with those symptoms. "Heart palpations, shortness of breath, lightning flashes, not possible to operate until we figure all that out," he said.

He pointed out on the recent November 9th blood work and the fine print disclaimer at the bottom on the last page. It says (translated into English for me) that even though you don't test positive on this blood test for Lyme bacteria, *it doesn't mean that you don't have it*. He further added his own commentary to the matter that this is some new writing they now include with all negative Lyme tests. "Look at the one from seven years ago," he said, "There's no possibility left open for that potential with their conclusions back then. We changed our thinking a few years ago."

Great I thought. I had to wait seven years before they would consider I might have Lyme disease even though nothing showed up on the blood work. I wondered how that thinking came about. That one little obscure line at the end of the recent 5-page blood report combined with my described symptoms over the past seven years stopped any possibility of going ahead with my knee surgery. That was this Surgeon's legal, ethical, and clinical full stop to not pull the trigger on surgery. The medical establishment could now hold the opinion I actually had Lyme bacteria swimming around inside me, just that they couldn't find it. Dr. Halverstadt already told me as much in September. At least it was nice to get these French Doctors' confirmation, but by then I was 100% percent into the Lyme camp anyway because of my obvious multiple symptoms driving me into a grave.

What next, and what to do? He picked up his digital Dictaphone and like an MSF field commander, rapid fired at least five minutes of monologue in French into his recorder. I got the drift of it loud and clear. He was describing all my Lyme symptoms and directing his comments to the

University of Limoges Lyme specialist group for full-blown testing by their best people who know Lyme. He said that's my next stop. Limoges University Medical System for more advanced Lyme testing.

Then It Got Even Worse

At this point, I'm not rattled by his professional opinion because I've got a holistic program killing off my Lyme bacteria and reams of current stem cell research at my back. It's not like I'm mentally defenseless at this point. And, I've been on the holistic sauce for almost two weeks and it seems to be doing something beyond creating expensive colored urine. One month ago, I would've been devastated with this Doctor's news.

So it was finally time to pop the 64-dollar question before I went out the door. I asked him about stem cell treatment and what he thought about stem cell cartilage re-growth.

I'd been lying low to ask that question directly to him for almost a month. Once I got deeper into the Regenexx daily blog flow and their periodic webinars, to me, it's a mandatory question that must be asked and answered during every orthopedic pre-surgery meeting today.

I like this doctor and sincerely respect his professional ability, but I didn't like his short shrift attitude about stem cell therapy. He said it doesn't work. It's unproven and not a consideration for my knee. Case closed, end of discussion. I knew I had crossed a boundary and knew when to call it quits. He told us his verbal report would find it into the system in a week or so and I'd be on my way to Limoges University Medicine for some high-powered testing.

I left his office with one indelible mental point from that

meeting. He's of the professional opinion that Stem cell therapy won't help my knee one iota. Same conclusion by my local GP a month ago, but yet the Doctors in Denver have performed their stem cell treatment on 23,500 patients as I write this passage December 18, 2015 . . . and they're picking up steam fast according to their blog site.

How about the guy in the Irish pub who got offered the stem cell option for his debilitating hip troubles in Limoges, France by the orthopedic clinic who did his titanium hip replacement? In addition to this pub guy's glowing comments about his incredibly rapid recovery at the 10-day marker, he did mention right *after* his surgery, he searched, *hip replacements with metal implants.* He was quite surprised to learn that micro bits of metal will wear off over time and can infect the blood. That bit of knowledge disturbed him considerably, but as he rationalized, "I've probably only got ten years left to live anyway." The old fatalist logic solves all, I thought. We timber cutters had a catch all phrase for every problem on earth, from bad food in camp, to bad breath, to bad government in Ottawa: "Fifty years from now, it won't make a fucking bit of difference." Meaning we'll all be dead by then anyhow, so why sweat the small stuff.

Maybe the gentleman in the bar is right: We're all dead someday anyway, does it matter when we get there? Individual taste and preference I suppose but I like the long scenic route myself. I find living kind of fun and I'm sticking with that philosophy until it isn't.

This again is the link to the stem cell Doctors in Denver. Regenexx

Where is the truth, Dear Reader? Where is the truth . . . ? I'll tell you the truth: It's whatever we want to believe and act upon. That's the truth. We're all headed where our minds take us . . . pure and simple. You may be wondering, "How did Jim feel after that pre-surgery meeting?" Let me reverse the tables. How would you have felt after that meeting?

Ambivalence? Superiority? Arrogance? Confusion? Fear? Mixed Emotions?

Keep reading and you'll find out soon enough because here is what went through my mind in a flash from the short walk between the surgeon's office and our car parked down the street.

Rewinding The Tapes

I rewound my mental tapes back eight weeks, back to the point when I was virtually clueless to all that's written on these previous 152 pages.

At that point in time eight weeks ago, without a doubt, I would've been elated that I was off to Limoges for study of my symptoms, and would've thought that finally this Lyme disease will be identified and I'll get on with their modern cure with the latest drugs or something effective to get rid on this chronic fatigue and fuzzy brain that's getting worse as the months drag by. End of story for the Lyme problem and then I can get on with the standard basic mechanical knee job. Easy peasy, nice and easy. That's what I would've thought eight weeks ago with this December 16th news. Hooray, hooray!

I would've been thinking how great is this? I now officially get the disabled car window sticker until the knee job is completely healed, Limoges and Périgueux will take care of everything in fine French style. Chatty nurses, wonderful doctors, chauffeured taxi service to Limoges and back, all paid for by insurance. What's not to like about this program?

Back then I had no clue that current medical thinking is

to attack those Lyme spirochetes with triple strength antibiotics for a minimum six to eight weeks and when that doesn't get it, then try again, and once again with IV antibiotics for twelve months if necessary or until yeast begins to ooze out of every body pore and skin sloughs off the lips. I had no clue what a year of antibiotic treatment can do to a person and would probably still be stuck with those spirochetes lurking in the deeps no matter how much antibiotic treatment they tried to throw at the problem. Back then, I didn't know that Lyme can appear to have been nicely all killed off, but then to everybody's surprise, the symptoms can pop right back months later . . . like those gophers in *Caddy Shack*.

Only later, after a long depressing wait to cure Lyme disease might I learn that Lyme was most likely eating away at the rest of my joints, my brain and my soul just like syphilis does. I didn't know any of this eight weeks ago. No . . . that bit of revelation may not have arrived into my consciousness until next summer while I'd still be waiting for the green light on surgery.

But I did know all these things when I went into my appointment yesterday. I did know about all the post-surgery complications and chronic pain that can plague a TKR recipient for years.

All I knew and believed two months ago is that these great French doctors were going to fix any problems I had with Lyme disease and my knees would work like brand new.
When I walked out the door of that clinic on December 16th after that doctor said there's no hope for my knees except surgery, but we have to wait until we figure out your Lyme symptoms, I never felt better in my life.

I'll tell you why I never felt better in my life . . . That

Doctor didn't know that at six in the morning that very same morning, I tested myself. I needed to make sure I'm not in some kind of delusional state praying to the Teasel god every morning and experiencing some sort of miracle in my mind, but not in reality. Dear Reader, I'm a no-bullshit, fucking hard nose timber cutter from way back and got this far in life by believing in just about everything and anything, but always faithfully living with stone cold reality.

That morning of Wednesday, December 16, 2015 at 6:00 a.m., in the dark, I lit out of the house with the dog on a leash, and no walking stick. I marched up to our mailbox and the bowser did his business. From the driveway, I turned left and out into the dark where I walked the entire 500-meter circuit in our field. Up one fence line, across the back line and down the backstretch to the driveway and home. That's over 800 meters of walking.

At 8:00 a.m., I slipped behind the wheel of our Renault Scenic and drove with my wife to Périgueux. We parked a block down a hill from the clinic and walked uphill to my appointment without a cane or the birch stick. After our meeting where I learned that my x-rays revealed that bone-on-bone knee joint to be a stage four basket case, I reversed the journey home, walked the dog to the same mail box, plus the 500-meter field circuit, and thanked my lucky stars I had visited Dr. Halverstadt in September, found Dr. Glidden in October, and Dr. Storl and the German teasel producers in November . . . and was on the whole protocol for twelve days when I left the Surgeons office December 16th.

Two weeks ago, I could have done none of that combined walking activity. No mailbox walk, no 500-meter circuit in the field, no driving to Périgueux, and no hill walk up to the clinic . . . times two. On top of that, two weeks ago, my brain was firing off lightning flashes and I was depressed and felt old and broken. Hoisting a few half sacs of groceries out of the car was my strength and endurance limit. That was my condition two weeks ago, Dear Reader.

Yes, I believe in God and miracles. God absolutely had his part in all this, but so did I. Sort of like the old parable I reserve for hypocritical bible thumpers when they don't give us earthlings much credit in the process of these special situations. And I'm not just picking on the Bible. That goes for the Talmud, the Torah, the Quran, the Book of Mormon, the Bhagavad-Gita and all the rest of the books including the book of Betty Crocker.

Those books are all sacred texts meant to be revered and quietly studied and spoken of discretely, not shoved down our throats and gagged on like a pair of old dirty gym socks.

The Parable I Live By

The passing lady commented on our beautiful flower gardens and what a lovely gift God has brought us. I agreed heartily, but I did comment back, "You should have seen this rock pile when God had it all by himself!"

What I believe in most is the miracle of life, the miracle of nature and the miracle of the universe that I can see every night when I look up into the stars. If we study them and live closely with them in our heart, we'll find ourselves closer to God. He'll bring us gifts constantly. We just have to keep our eyes peeled.

The rest of all life's miracles fit somewhere in between those three realms and they're happening all the time. When a baby is born, when a butternut squash comes into harvest in October, when the winter solstice swings us back into advancing daylight for another six months which sustains all of life on earth, or when a GPS signal pings back and forth to an iPhone, in timed unison with a cesium atomic clock . . . these are miracles to me. Scoring a door buster new flat screen of Black Friday is a miracle too . . . for some I suppose.

My knee and my brain and my body and my spirit healing this rapidly in fourteen days, is a miracle too. I call it the miracle of life. That's how I felt walking out of that clinic in Périgueux. I felt like I'm a living fucking miracle on his way to recovery. I felt like Rocky Balboa prancing up the steps of the Philadelphia Court House prepared for the prize fight of his life. I felt like an underdog two weeks ago. On the morning of the 16th of December, I felt like a champion who was on a winning streak and was just getting warmed up for the second round of his life. That's how I felt leaving that office. Like a winner. Not a loser like the one I had felt like for the last seven years. "I'm in the fight of my life and totally ready for anything that comes my way," I thought. "Bring it on," I yelled inside me walking down that sidewalk back to the car from the surgeons office, "I'm fucking ready to fight anything out there because I have a universe of holistic natural healing backing up my body, my brain, and my spirit." That's how I felt . . . never mentally stronger in my entire life. Never stronger in my life.

I believe we must be aware, vigilant, and active . . . Not wary, just aware and proactive in all areas of our life, not just health . . . but like my grandmother said, "Jimmy Jam, your health is the most important thing you have. Take care of it."

I didn't feel a fist-pumping chest-thumping elation or arrogance as I walked out of that Périgueux clinic. I didn't feel angry, concerned, nervous or uncertain about the future. I felt very grateful. I felt very grateful as I walked out that door. I knew as I walked down that hill from the clinic in Périgueux, I'd publish this book and for the rest of my life, try to spread this message that our bodies can heal in holistic ways, if we believe and act upon that belief intelligently. That's what this story is all about: Proactive, intelligent holistic healing.

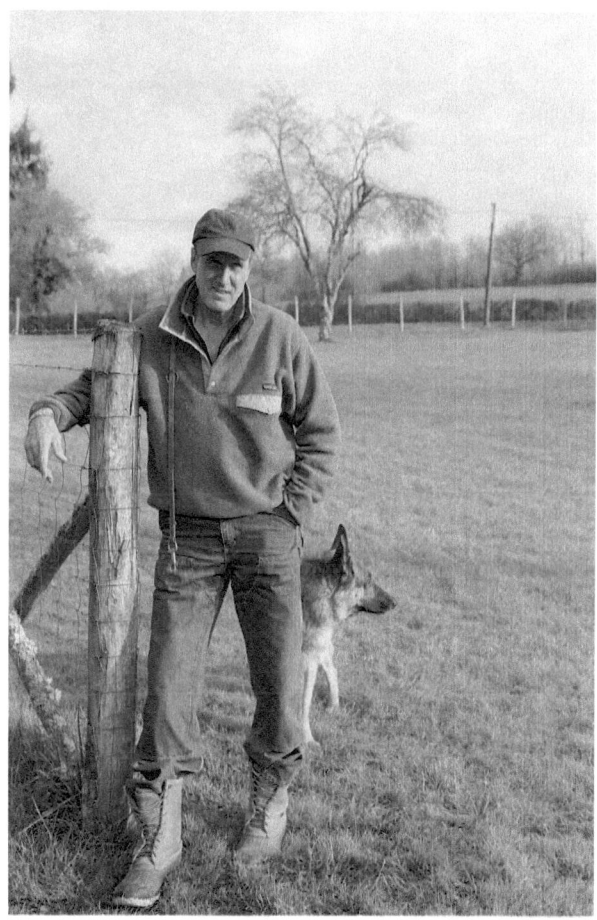

My 500-Meter Field Circuit, December 20, 2015

This is the start of my 500-meter field circuit. The same one I walked in the dark on December 16th, 2015. This has become my benchmark of knee joint improvement. These pictures show the entire field circuit. For the time being, until my knee gets better, my plan is to minimize any walking to let the cartilage grow back without grinding it all off before it has a chance to improve.

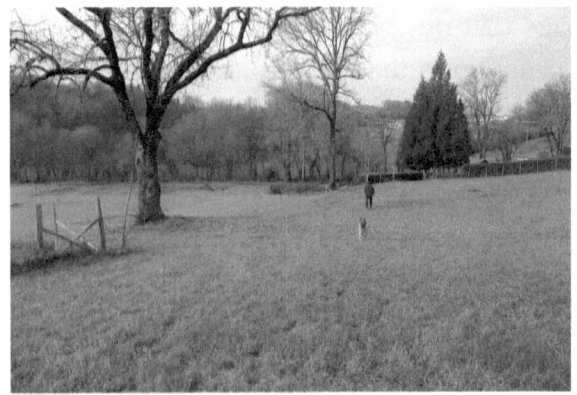

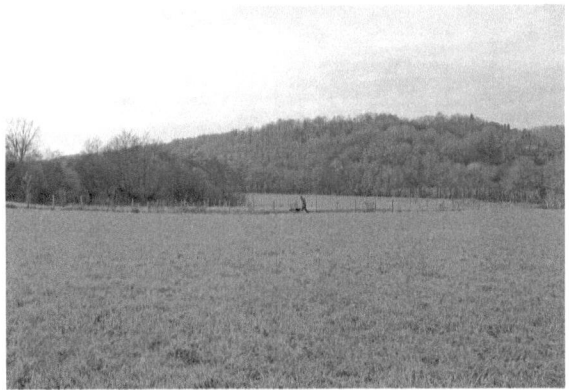

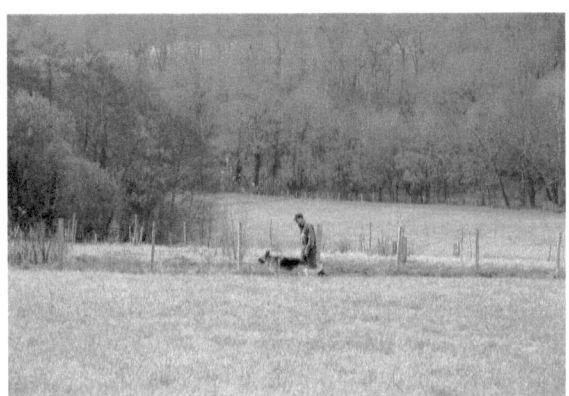

My 500-Meter Field Circuit, December 20, 2015

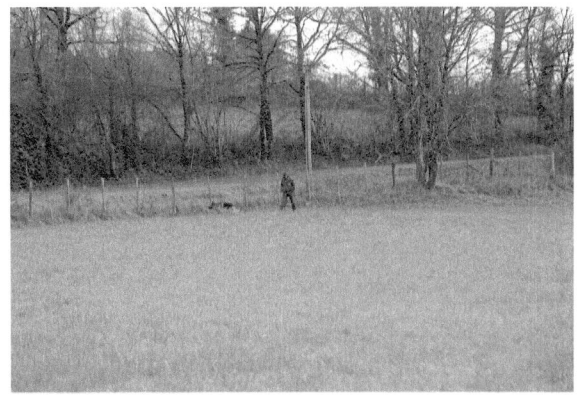

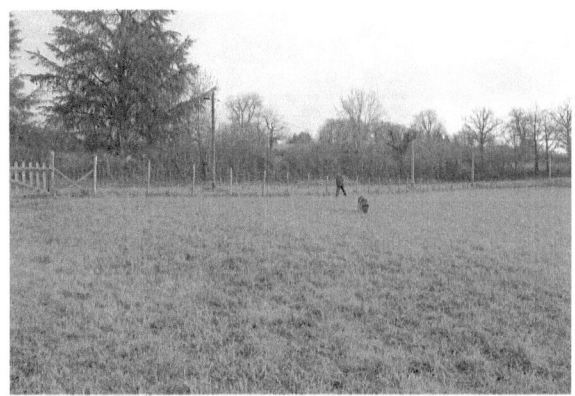

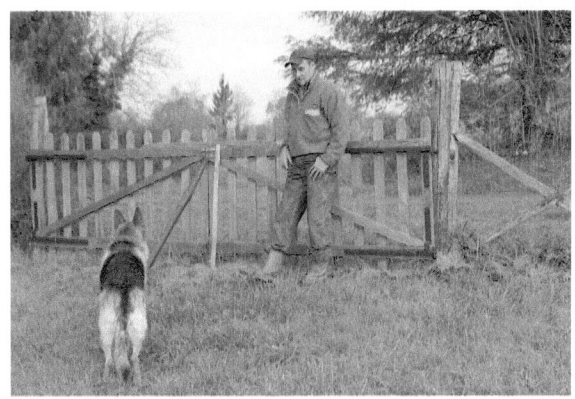

My 500-Meter Field Circuit, December 20, 2015

Chapter 10:
It's Getting Dark Inside

Tuesday, December 22, 2015, 6:25 a.m.
Day 16 On The Full Cartilage & Lyme Protocol
Day 18 On The Teasel
31 Days Since Beginning This Journal

I need to broach the subject of vulgarity. I believe it's a very important topic to analyze at this juncture in the healing process because as you can read, a certain coarseness is breaking out. Almost like a fever.

Coarseness isn't me. It's not welcome among the circles of friends, colleagues, and strangers I want to associate with. No more than I like to hang out in close quarters with phlegmy coughing sick people. Vulgarity used constantly can be like a sickness. It, to me, underlies something's not correct. Something out of kilter. The more they curse, the farther out of balance the person is wobbling off center. Some cussy people are like a dangerous human top spinning out of control putting themselves and their loved ones in emotional danger. I believe it's our job not to judge these people as they come unglued but to stand back out of harm's way from all their flying toxic infective spittle as they express something troubling through their vulgarity.

"What is the source of these eruptions . . . these fevers of vulgarity?" I ask with fascination . . . starting with me!

Maybe it's the spirochete debris pilling up in my brain

waiting for the next ride out the door and I'm thoroughly pissed off the garbage truck is stuck in the back alley . . . metaphorically of course, at a very deep subconscious level. Who knows for sure.

I like that visual . . . *Toxic infective spittle*. That's my new definition of vulgar utterances: Toxic infective spittle.

But just wait a minute! Is it always toxic? Is it always tasteless? Is it always spittle? Is it always insensitive, overreaching behaviors? The following over-the top caricature sketch is offered here to be pondered. This is a serious character study, but please skip this entire next paragraph if you're sensitive to completely tasteless vulgarity. It's offered here only to illustrate my point in the extreme. Some crude logger might pepper his conversation with even more color, but his heart would be no less loving and sincere.

Here is a scene of a he-man logger who explodes in an ecstatic high fidelity roaring bellow, like a raging bull in testosterone super overdrive, beaming with warm fatherly pride to all his timber cutting buddies down at the bar, yelling at the top of his lungs after a few too many beers and when asked how his wife is now doing with the birthing cycle of life

"I'm so crazy fucking happy, she delivered two beautiful twins yesterday in that beautiful fucking hospital while I was right there beside her. Fuck me gently, it was so fucking beautiful I couldn't fucking believe it!"

And then these intimate logging buddies all high five together with this cussing beast of a man, kiss him on his head and all get stinking ass drunk because this beast and his wife had been trying to have children for the past ten years, and this lonely fatherless timber cutter is the last one on the crew to begin his family and continue the cycle of his life that he and his wife so desperately wanted. What if this is the happiest day of this beast's life and he wants to celebrate it with his most intimate friends?

Is that outburst… pustulent social discourse? Is that toxic tasteless vulgarity? Is that a choice of words that indicates some mysterious deep malaise? No, I believe, that type of vulgar outburst isn't vulgar at all. I believe in this case it's a sign of deep love among a bunch of tough little boys who have no other way to say I love you among emotionally insular men who all care for each other deeply.

Maybe, sometimes, vulgarity is a person's passageway into a more intimate world. Maybe vulgarity is my passageway into a more intimate world. I'll have to back track and look at it from that perspective. Maybe my deeper truth lies hidden in my vulgarity. Maybe when a person let's some cuss words fly, we should pay special attention because that's their most important expression of feeling, and they're trying to reach out. Maybe we should be thankful for vulgarity, because at least people are honestly expressing themselves. Vulgarity might be an important component in human communication and relationship development. So now, let me advance and expand my definition of vulgar speech considering the beast-scene just described.

Jim's New World Dictionary Definition Of Vulgarity

Vulgar free speech is no more than toxic vocal human spittle when the underlying voice of the speaker is grounded in fear, hate, anger or malice, and it may indicate a deep malaise likely hidden to both the speaker and the recipient of the spittle.

On The Other Hand

Vulgar free speech can also be equated to pure human goodness and joy when the underlying voice of the speaker is grounded in love and the speaker has a deep desire to express that love, but is inhibited to fully express himself to the recipient in a more conventional manner of speaking. Likely, both the speaker and the recipient can feel that bond of love but are unable to acknowledge it openly.

Dear Reader, I believe most vulgarity lands somewhere between these two wide margins of social behavior of love and anger. Our job as the recipient listener is to cipher the underlying reasons for vulgar outbursts in the first place. That's what I'm trying to figure out with my slide into this interior darkness of speech creeping over these pages. I ask where does it come from. Is the Teasel breaking down some unseen barriers more than just those nasty spirochetes?

And here might be my dog's simple rejoinder to all this vulgarity discourse if he could chime into the conversation:

What you say to me, Dear Master, isn't nearly as important as how you feel about what you say to me, since I don't understand a single word of your language anyway. It's the tone Dear Master, it's the tone that belies the truth of your every spoken word. Sing me your music of kindness and I will respond. Sing me your music of hostility and I will also respond. One I will stay, the other I will leave you. One I will love you, the other, you may never know how I feel because I will be gone from your toxic world.

Sometimes I think dogs understand our human communication better than we humans understand each other.

Back To My Brewing Stew

I believe the flare up of my truculent vulgarity is a sign. Like a boil that shows up on the skin, like a nice full yellow and reddish pustulent formation indicating that something is going on deeper inside the body. My vulgarity boil is probably indicating toxicity and unhappy cells. And when that boil erupts because of too much pressure, the toxins are ready to come out and the body ready to heal. Cursing is like that I think. With each cussy utterance, a bit of human resident toxicity flows out into the room at large. We know the boorish types where we need to don a hazmat suit to stay safe. I might have been one of the boorish types in my past. I hope not, but I probably was a time or two.

I believe vulgar eruptions can also be indicators of the healing process-taking place. A release of verbal eruptions is a good thing in the healing process. I think it's better to expel mental pus out of the system than hold it in and exacerbate the underlying condition it belies. I believe I've come down with a fever. A general vulgar malaise. Let's call it "Teasel Fever Vulgaritus Expandus-Contractus." Meaning my vulgarity seems to come and go. It would be nice if it left for good.

Wednesday, December 23, 2015, 8:12 a.m.

I had a nice special challis session earlier and added a short little addendum to the ritual. I believe all sincere rituals should have a tiny bit of secrecy to them. A secret bond between the true believer and the Big Guy up there. Like witnessing the Masonic secret hand shake. It happens so fast you might think you observed it, but not really. There's always that little bit of good mystery to ancient rituals. I'm like that with mine.

I've prayed in the Kings Chamber of the Great Pyramid of Giza. I've prayed at the Sacred Alter of ancient Akhenaton in Karnak. I've prayed in the Great Cathedral of Notre Dame and at least a few hundred other churches, temples and altars around the world. I've prayed in the Mormon Tabernacle in Salt Lake City, and prayed among the twirling sacred Sufis in Fez, Morocco at my birthday party. I've prayed from mountaintops and prayed in the silence of ancient giant cedar groves, in hidden Virgin Forests. I've prayed a lot in my life, but I can tell you this, the Teasel Ritual is pretty special for me. It's right up there with the best and getting better each day. I like people. I like different cultures. I like to experience others' sincere spirituality. Maybe I can learn something from them. Maybe some of it'll rub off on me. Who knows.

I believe I've been unbelievably fortunate these past few weeks. I believe God has lined up all the healing billiard balls for me, and now it's up to me to try and run the table. He has done his part, now I have to make something out of this rock pile in front of me and turn it into a garden of vibrant health. That was my Teasel message today, but it's not going to be simple. My recent outbursts of vulgarity tell me not every day will be easy. That was my message in meditation today: It's not going to be simple.

Laguna Beach Syndrome

In my entire life, I've never felt a burning compulsion to write anything on paper, save one time. This journal is only the second time in almost thirty years.

I've written probably an average amount of business and personal material like most active people, but none of that material was ever in the category of first order compulsory dictate. Almost thirty years ago, it happened, but never again. This journal, to me, is approaching that compulsory category. Let me explain.

Many years ago, I was walking our dog on a ridge top high above Laguna Beach, California overlooking the Pacific Ocean. Out of nowhere, a bolt of inspiration hit my brain. When the dog and I got back to our rented house a little later, I began to write. BIC pen on yellow legal lined paper, top to bottom, three pages, non-stop scribbling. It just flowed out of my brain, down the arm, into the pen onto the paper . . . like magic.

There was zero editing, or margin notes. The first words: "The other day" . . . to the last period, were all handwritten. I signed it, folded it up, sealed it into an envelope, looked up the Wall Street Journal's address from a newspaper lying in the house, and sent it to the Chief Editor's attention. I noticed Dr. Kissinger had just penned some feature article about something in that day's edition.

Now please understand this was April, 1987. Long before the internet and Microsoft Word. Every word I wrote that day, hit my brain in a micro flash during that dog walk and it stuck word for word, as I wrote to the editor on that yellow scratch pad. I didn't think. I just wrote, and it flowed onto the paper. That's pretty much how these pages occur for the past couple of weeks. There's no outline, no pre-thought, like . . . oh, that would be a cute title. *Farting at Lake Helen* should get their attention . . . I just write.

What you're reading for the past 166 pages was written without forethought. It just flowed. I feel like I'm a reporter assigned to cover a story at Times Square after my boss instructed me to just write about whatever shows up on the street for the next six months. Just stand there, observe and write. If the Macy's Day parade flows by, report it. If the New Year's Eve Ball gets dropped, report it. If a terrorist asks me to hold his bomb belt while he uses the toilet in Starbucks on his way to blow up the subway, I report it.

For me personally, as I'm writing these pages, I'm out of the story. I'm the reporter on this guy *Jim* trying to heal himself. I'm waiting on the street corner of his brain, and stuff just pops up and I write about Jim, like I did for the Wall Street Journal almost thirty years ago. That's how all these zany chapter titles are birthed. That's how all this narrative is birthed. It just pops up as I'm observing this healing process of a guy named Jim Lindl.

So if you're shocked to learn that my little letter on yellow scratch pad paper got that editor's attention, you're not as shocked as I was.

I about fell over when the phone rang, and that someone was interested in my little 3-page bolt out of the blue. She was the assistant editor to THE Big Guy. She said, "HE wants to run it immediately because of its timeliness." I asked, "How soon?" She said, "As soon as they could get some art work sketched up to accompany my writing."

"Holy Corona," I thought.

Then she went on to ask if she could change some punctuation. I told her she could rewrite the whole bloody thing if she wanted. I was absolutely agog.

I never graduated from high school. I was an ADD/ADHD mess for too many years. I stuttered my way through grade school and couldn't speak my own name without stalling out in frustration on the playground with the other kids, and yet today, I was on the phone with the *Wall Street Journal* in New York City!

We talked while she edited on the phone. She was lightning fast. She got my message loud and clear on those three yellow pages before she typed them into her own computer. I mean she must have read more high sermons and more unadulterated philosophical nonsense, like my ramblings on vulgarity, than most. She later told me she read more than 175 submissions each month of unsolicited verbiage like mine. How she ever weeded out my dinky submission in that reading stack I do not know but probably because it was the only one ever handwritten on yellow legal paper. She must have thought who would be so audacious to send in crab-handed chicken scratch to the WSJ Editor in Chief.

As my shock was wearing off, I began thinking this is big league serious. I was talking to the assistant editor of the WSJ, the most prestigious business newspaper in the world, with the highest circulation of any newspaper on the entire planet. This paper is the great brain engine of modern day capitalism and political economic discourse for the entire world and she thought my unsolicited submission was cleverly breezy, satirical but not arrogant, an incisive artistic cut to the *essence* of Federal Reserve policy at the time. Yes, indeed. It was the chairman of the Federal Reserve and its policies of money printing that I was indirectly addressing in my satirical screed of truth and fiction.

I explained to the world why the stock market was levitating like a magic carpet. It was all about funny money euphemistically called *Liquidity Injections*. These Federal Mandarins, unelected by anybody, but owned and ruled by a few private big banks all tied together through the BIS in Switzerland, acted like some modern day economic stem cell doctors . . . Add a shot here, add a shot there, and everything in the economy will grow just ducky. Little did anyone know that it was all fairy dust they were injecting that would grow into a worldwide systemic cancer in thirty years. I knew about this cancer causing fairy dust, and wasn't afraid to write about it and tell the world. The Federal Reserve was launching a really cool party back then, but so was Jim Jones in Jonestown until the Kool-Aid kicked in . . . but how to get such a message out? With a dash of satire, Dear Reader. She was reading a profound truth smothered in satire that flowed onto those three yellow pages, which were telegraphed directly into my brain on that ridge top in Southern California.

I obliquely pontificated it was all about printed money from the Federal reserve and not good luck from outer space that was the rocket propellant blasting the stock market and rare art prices into the stratosphere. This type of mainstream monetary nonsense is plain vanilla gospel today that everybody knows who owns an ATM card. Not a big revelation today. Even in mid-stream of this grand super cycle of contrived monetary design, one ornery vice president even professed that *deficits don't matter*. What a silly goose he was to say such a preposterous thing . . . yes, deficits do matter! They absolutely do matter.

Without the funny money Fed deficits, recycled through Petrodollar accounts, none of this monetary charade could ever continue past next Tuesday morning and yet today . . . we've transcended into the spiritual realm of funny money printing. The abuse, the suffering and the squandering are breathtaking to witness and our health is impacted by it all. It's called societal stress! Societal disorder. Societal dysfunction.

Our life and our very soul have been hacked and hijacked by this pernicious monetary system. This tired old abused Ship of State is creaking as the popping riveted seams are giving off serious malfunction signals. Are we heeding these critical signals? . . . or are we conveniently, collectively just ignoring them. We know the answer. It's obvious.

Back then, this truth was considered deep thinking: The Fed's mystery monetary liquidity power driving the Dow Jones average past 2,000. How quaint a Dow at 2,000 is today and people getting excited about that back then. The world was just getting warmed up for the main act. What was started back then, affects all of us today with Social Security and Medicare going broke as just two prime examples of insiders madness to build an empire on the back of Mid-East fueled and recycled dollar-based debt!

It's endless fairy dust wealth creation until it isn't. Like those coastal virgin forests were destined to last forever, until they were all gone. That's exactly where Medicare is headed in my lifetime. Social Security as well. Poof . . . Gone. What a surprise! "Where did it all go?" we'll collectively ask one day.

This whole game is about keeping the gravy train on the tracks for a few more years. I saw that bright light far down the monetary tunnel thirty years ago. How quaint. But know this, as sure as the sun will rise tomorrow morning: Understanding and following this long running Fed cycle of monetary liquidity madness is about as important as following the latest Bruce/Caitlyn, Caitlyn/Bruce glamour fashion . . . and they're both about an equal time wasting spectacle of the same magnitude, in my opinion. It's like the weather outside. We can't do a darn thing about *their* monetary policy so why worry. It's going to rain whether we like it or not.

But back then, it wasn't quaint. It was profound! Unbelievable how times have changed, in all things money related around the world. Those of us who are expecting a little something on the back end after a lifetime of hard work and tax contribution may be very surprised in the coming years. All of this impacts our health and we can't do a single thing about it but ponder and brood or change the channel on the flat screen to more pleasant scenery.

I could see it all coming thirty years ago but also knew it was unstoppable. Why unstoppable you ask? Because we are human and it's been all too much fun for us humans to continue driving our own cushy tour bus right over the cliff in willful delusion, while collectively thinking it would all nicely work out.

Brilliant observation and analysis it was back then, I must admit, but I knew who the true author was. I never have believed for a minute to this day that it was me who wrote those three yellow lined pages. I was like a radio receiver getting a message from outer space on that ridge top in California and my arm and hand converted that celestial radio beacon into intelligible meaning, like a stylus on a phonograph for us earthlings to understand. I was simply the message carrier for that day.

Yes, I do understand a couple of things about monetary policy, historical geopolitics, political economy, and empire building. But the timing of that spontaneous writing, clear, laden with a powerful-cloaked message, didn't originate in my brain. It came to me from a higher power. No other explanation is plausible. I've never written another worthwhile original thing since.

It was published, and I got invited to their offices, and later had lunch with them at the still standing World Trade Center. We talked about life, about the world. Theirs and mine. Totally different people in two totally different worlds drawn together in New York City by three simple hand written pages. That editor believed I had more wisdom in me to write . . . but about what? I didn't know what. It's been quite a long drought of inspiration these past thirty years.

Well, Dear Reader, I've never felt as compelled to write

about anything like I did that day in Laguna Beach until recently. That was the last time I felt that way until I began this journal 32 days ago. I don't think about what I'm writing here, I just write. My arm just moves. But lately I do feel like my radio receiver is turned back on again and somebody out there's trying to transmit into the darkest and deepest corners of my very soul.

Chapter 11:
Full Moon Rising

Christmas Eve
Thursday, December 24, 2015, 3:56 p.m.
Day 18 On The Full Cartilage & Lyme Protocol
Day 20 On The Teasel
33 Days Since Beginning This Journal

Today is turning out to be a rough day. Nine days since the Great *Green Mile* Blowout and the bull bellowing lion roaring ... then this afternoon, another blowout event swept over me that rhymed with the first one on the 15th of December. Different, but yet the same: mild coughing, gentle farting, a 107°F shower and major plop-plop-plop into the ten-ring. Not a dark mud pie like last time, more like a soft light chocolate cream smoothie dispensed out of a machine.

Abbreviated notes for now because I'm still shaking off a massive headache. Just got up from a deep two-hour sleep after the blow out. Likely, the first full Herxheimer (Herx) reaction that all the experts suggest can occur during Teasel Lyme Battles. They suggest it'll occur about the two-week marker. Mine was just about three weeks on the nose.

Was able to put an early log onto the fire and do the Teasel Ritual. Got a message while meditating: Cycles are everywhere including the healing I'm going through. Then the Chapter 11 title popped into the writing. Today is a full Moon on Christmas Eve. It'll be another 17 years before the next full moon on this date. Interesting to me the number 17. I haven't a clue about numerology, but plenty of people study these things very seriously.

The number 17 is a constant recurring number for me ever since I waited on the 17th floor in my apartment in Edmonton for back surgery in December, 1976. I walked out of my back surgery hospitalization 39 years ago today, Christmas Eve in the late afternoon. That number 17 has been present all my life at important junctures: April 17, the first day I started work after graduating from university. The day I quite that first job three years later, to the day, April 17, and took a new direction. My wife's birthday. The day myself, a few others and two venture capitalists founded our new vitamin company, March 17, 1993, and hundreds of times over the past 39 years the number 17 has just shown up. When all the rooms are sold out in a hotel with just one left . . . you guessed it . . . number 17 is often the one waiting. This type of full moon won't reappear again until I'm 80 years old . . . in 17 years. $1+7=8$, $8\times10=80$.

Ten is the perfect universal number because it ends everything in numerology, but also begins everything in numerology. Ten is the ending, it's the last number of everything and then it begins all over again with . . . $1+0=1$, which is the beginning of everything, the first number of them all . . . and on and on and on . . .

One night I rode down Interstate 80 between Sacramento and San Francisco with a Rosicrucian at the wheel of his Mercedes Benz for a few hours. In the quiet darkness of that ride, the driver said, "Everything can be explained in the numbers." He talked just like I wrote above for hours and after a while, it actually made sense. It was all very convoluted and technical. Fascinating actually. He knew his stuff. That as twenty some years ago. Today I haven't a clue about numerology and that quiet late night ride down Interstate 80 is lost in the fog of time.

Maybe my knees won't heal up until I'm eighty years old! Who knows.

Right now, it's back to bed. I'm pretty sick. This is hopefully a good sign. A good turning point. I haven't a clue if this 17 and full moon business means anything in numerology or biology, anthropology or geology, astrology or proctology. But I'll take note of today since I do believe today, the day before Christmas, could be some kind of doorway into my future that leads to better health. It did 39 years ago on Christmas Eve when I came home from that Edmonton hospital all strung out on Valium and painkillers. I was destined to redirect my life back then. Maybe I am again today. Who knows. Thirty-nine, $3+9=12$, $1+2=3$, three is the key because it can represent the Sacred Trinity of Life, Light and Love, or Father, Son, and Holy Ghost or Body, Mind and Spirit.

Take your pick but I think they're all the same, just different ways of expressing the three part system that powers everything around us including the entire universe we see at night up to the stars and beyond to the boundaries of time and space, which are unbounded because it's all built in the mind of God . . . which knows no limits just as our human ability to think and dream and believe all the way back to God himself is limitless. That's how, I believe, we humans are inescapably and inseparably all hooked together . . . through our mind which leads us directly to our heart and soul, which interconnects every living thing in the universe together with each other and with God. God, to me, is like the power plant of the Universe and we creatures of life light and love all radiate with variable luminosity reflecting life's beautiful harmony or its darkness and anger and dysfunction, depending how well our wires are connected to the main transmission line back to God, the source of all energy and love. Belief and meditation upon a supreme power force opens up the possibilities of God. I believe that a fifth source that scientists are so desperately looking for . . . is hiding in plain sight. I believe it surrounds us.

I believe, that sincere belief in anything good we want to happen in our lives will happen, because of the transmission line back to God, to this ultimate power source, to gain our energy and our spiritual brightness of life, light and love. That I know is a possibility for sure, because it's worked for me my entire life. Things happen when we truly believe they're going to happen. They just do.

You have no doubt heard all the timeless refrains: "If we believe, we can conceive." "If there's a will, there's a way." "As a man thinketh, so he becomes." "We reap what we sow." "If we ask, we receive." And on and on and on. Dear Reader, I believe everything we need is always hiding in plain sight waiting to be plucked off the shelf. We just have to ask intelligently with respect, humility, and gratefulness. Stuff will just show up, but we need to do our part and keep our eyes peeled or we can miss the gifts staring us right in the face.

Time for some deep rest and more healing. I'm drifting off to get a better connection with that transmission line hooked to the main power plant. I never want to get unplugged for too long.

These last few paragraphs, written on Christmas Eve, 2015, just before I turned in for the night, will hopefully all make sense one day.

Chapter 12: Reflection, Review & More Reflection

Sunday, December 27, 2015, 9:06 p.m.
Day 21 On The Full Cartilage & Lyme Protocol
Day 23 On The Teasel
11 Days Since The Périgueux Surgery Meeting
35 Days Since Beginning This Journal

This is a good time to do an overall review. That was the message I got during the Teasel meditation on December 25 when this title came to me. I've not felt particularly bright for a few days so I spent the past two days reading, resting, healing, and adding in some of the photos into the previous 178 pages. In that process, a few words were added or changed. A few sentences were added or changed. A few thoughts were added or changed, all for the purpose of clarity. Everything else remains as in the original except where the heat from a few verbal cayenne passages needed to be hosed down . . . and a couple of toxic paragraphs were hosed off the pages for good.

This chapter isn't supposed to be about spontaneous narrative. This chapter is supposed to be a review with critical thinking about the past few months. This chapter is supposed to be a reflection of the healing process during the past few days and weeks and months since embarking on this life changing journey. There should be no ridge top down loads in this section.

From this analysis, resolve to continue this path or possibly make some course corrections, should be evident by the conclusion of this chapter. We'll see.

The seven questions I ask myself at this day twenty-three juncture on this holistic Nutritional -Teasel Protocol:

1) How am I doing? Compared to what?
2) Am I improving? Compared to what?
3) Is this the best course of action? Compared to what?
4) Is there more I should be doing? Compared to what?
5) Have I become complacent in my study and analysis? Compared to what?
6) Am I prepared to shift gears if pertinent information presents itself? Yes or no? Why yes? Why not?
7) Am I avoiding anything obvious? If yes, why?

Regarding Question 1

I've heard it said from several chiropractors over the years there's a natural God given healing sequence in the overall human body that goes like this: *Worst First, Inside Out, Top Down*. This physiological priority is how the body triages its healing sequence if there are multiple items to fix and repair, given the body's autonomic inherent survival imperative, and its system limitations to create the necessary energy and spiritual/mental balance to gain full recovery back to optimal health.

In other words, things get fixed that are the most important for survival . . . one at a time. It's like the total combination of maladies in Jim Lindl's body are all standing in line in the Doctor's reception room, waiting their turn to get attended to by the body's healing power. The Doctor decides what needs fixing first. In holistic thinking, the body will figure that sequence out automatically and decide what to fix first.

Here is my list of symptoms and stuff going on from the time period about June, 2015 up to the day I started this self-healing protocol December 4th, 2015, twenty-three days ago. I've been very cognizant of this worst first healing business since the day I began . . . waiting to see what was going to happen first . . . good or bad.

The Last Six Months: Physical Lethargy, Debilitating Fatigue, & Diminishing Strength

These would set in mid-afternoon every day. Our little farm has a myriad of different rural elements to keep it all ship shape and humming. These daily activities and continuing projects were never considered chores or work to me because I love physical work and keeping busy with most any type of activity.

Over eight years ago, when we bought this place everything to me around here was in the, "I love doing this, what a great life" category.

Seven years ago, after I began needing the birch stick to walk, some of the activity here had moved into the, "This is work" category.

Slowly, more and more things I use to love doing became necessary chores just to keep this place running. Cutting grass was one of the first I noticed had become tedious, if not unpleasant.

Later yet, most things began to weigh down on me like a burden to keep it all going. At about this juncture I began to feel old. This period was probably about three years after the tick bite.

By the Summer of 2014, we stated hiring occasional help because I just couldn't keep up any more. Things like cutting up trees and brush, moving piles of rocks, climbing ladders to cut vines on the house. Things began to be neglected. Little things like fully cleaning up after a project and tiding things up around the house. I began making excuses why things didn't matter anymore: Like vacuuming the car interior, which always attracts dirt, twigs, grass, leaves and bugs from around an active organic veggie farm. "We live on a farm," became my justification for letting things slip. Little by little, it was a normal downward spiral into old age, I thought.

The barn got disorganized more than usual. I made less frequent trips to Périgueux . . . maybe once every six to eight weeks, instead of twice monthly.

My wife began making city runs herself. I quit going to our local outdoor festive Saturday morning market. I told my neighbors I've become a hermit . . . and I was.

Yard work, gardening, and general work motivation ended mid-day. Work beyond this time took a determined push, almost a desperate will to get some things done. Like taking the garbage in the car up to the recycle bins twice per week. Giving the dog an outdoor bath. Clipping the dog's toenails Things were slowly getting neglected.

Muscle strength had been diminishing for years since the tick bite. By June, 2015 I kept saying to my wife or anybody that would listen that I can't lift this or that, because I have to protect my bad back from the surgery 40 years ago. Places like the plant nursery in Périgueux, the Farmers Co-Op in Thiviers, or the local hardware supply store. I let others lift things into the car, like sacks of peat moss, sacks of decorative stone or a lawn mower that needed repair. I couldn't put them into the car, but yet my older neighbors did all this type of work effortlessly.

My wife always made the grocery runs herself, packing and loading everything into the car at the store. I always unloaded the car at home but for the past two years I could barely even do that. She could lift more easily than I could for the past two years. By June, I couldn't even chase that stinking badminton birdie I had bought for us to play badminton on our lawn. I thought, "Geez Louise, most people don't ever retire until they're 65 years old, then they go off to play golf, hike the Grand Canyon, go on an African Safari, take up a martial art, or run a marathon . . . and I couldn't even chase a stinking badminton birdie." Something was very wrong, I thought.

My work activity and motivation level devolved over the last seven years: From, I love doing this . . . to, I want to do this . . . to, do I have to do this? . . . to, I'll do it later, . . . to, I'm getting too old for this . . . to, I can't do this anymore . . . to, It doesn't matter anymore . . . to September, 2015, when I didn't care what happened because I was too tired to worry. We have a lot of older people in our commune of 274 people and I thought, now I'm one of them.

During August, while building our new natural river fed swimming pool, I was required to direct our contractors during this 5-week project. I like to work with tools. I've always worked with all kinds of tools. I'm good with certain tools. Tools are something that are part of my life. I've invented and designed a new unique power tool for STIHL, an iconic German Company, who'll sell them into the worldwide marketplace. I know tools.

During this pool construction project, I'd sometimes find myself transfixed in a slow motion haze trying to assist the crew in certain elements of this project. They were very respectful of my condition but could see something was keeping me in a slow drift. Surreal for me. I was engaged into the job mentally, but couldn't function except sometimes in bizarre slow motion. Not slow in thought as much as slow in physical motion. I blamed it all on my sore knee. At the time, I had no idea I had Lyme disease.

One particular day in early September, I was at a portable workbench on the pool site with a skill saw, a belt sander and a power drill, fabricating a double thick oak door twenty-four inches square by 3.5 inches thick to be all nicely screwed together. Beautiful clear French white oak plank material all fastened together with long stainless steel wood screws. A wonderful little technical project for controlling the river flow into this concrete and stone lined river fed swimming hole. This type of technical futzing is my bailiwick.

This door should have taken me about an hour to measure, cut, bevel and assemble, and then sand smooth. In fact, it occupied my full capability from early morning until 3:00 p.m. Those Lyme corkscrew spirochetes working on the brain and the muscles must have been the cause. There's no other explanation that I can rationalize. Not my knee. I was standing in one spot, at that bench all day, doing nothing but struggle and drift along in a mental fog. That was the first week of September, 2015.

Bizarre, but at the time, I just thought I was an old man who ran out of timber. That little white oak door project went by in slow motion, with summer bugs buzzing around my head from the nearby slack river water, while I stared at the crew working as if they were powerful robots from some strange parallel universe. "If they weren't human robots," I thought, "Jim Lindl was certainly a broken down, tired mess."

Scenes like that happened all throughout this pool project. I usually work solo around this farm but during this 5-week project while I was in ultra-slow motion . . . and constantly compared myself to the work pace of one 45 year old cement mason and carpenter . . . I wondered what had happened to me as I watched him work? Why was I getting weak so fast?

It was on this pool project that I got a couple of good scares with my heart. Three or four times out of the blue, my heart would race up to almost 200 beats per minute and stay there for good twenty to thirty minutes. My breath would get short and I'd just lie down in the shade right in the middle of the job. I told the crew I was just a little tired, that everything was okay. I knew better. They just worked around me while I recovered.

Our household butane gas bottle, fuel for the stove in the kitchen, weighs 56 pounds full. Five years ago, I could easily carry a fresh full one 75 yards from the barn into the house in one hand. About three years ago I began using a wheelbarrow to get it into the kitchen and then eventually needed the wheelbarrow to carry the old empty one back out. These steel gas cylinders weigh 26 pounds empty and I didn't want to carry it by its handle back to the barn.

I used to carry a full armload of firewood in the crook of my arm into the house with another piece gripped by the fingers in the left hand, pushing the door open with my right foot. By December 4th, when I started this healing journey, I couldn't grip with my fingers the end of one single 10-pound piece of firewood in either my left of right hand. "I was just old," I thought.

All of these general work type activities stopped mid-September of 2015 because I was too weak. I thought it was entirely due to my back and neck out of adjustment. I was weak yes, but I thought it was also rapid aging causing the troubles. I hadn't a clue about anything related to Lyme bacteria at this point. Not until I traveled to California later.

Over the years I've had numerous friends and colleagues, and business associates die in their fifty's and early sixty's. But almost always it was cancer or a heart attack and usually pretty quick . . . 60 days to 16 months . . . but I had never known anybody who just withered from robust health into such a pathetic state of foggy, fuzzy mental helplessness over a few years' time without having a stroke or an industrial accident or something identifiable. I had no clue it was Lyme bacteria until I went to California mid-September for help. I made that California trip because I knew I had nowhere else to turn. I had run out of timber.

This was roughly my general *physical* state up to December 4th, 2015, before beginning this healing process.

The mental state from June to December, 2015 was, "Hold That Thought." My mental state for me wasn't as easily defined. My wife noticed it coming a long time ago, not so much me at the time.

The biggest thing my wife claims is that I became chronically forgetful. I never did see that part of my mental deterioration. From her perspective, it was pronounced.

What I had totally lost, was my ability to multi-task, even the most simple things. For example, if you were talking to me in the car, I'd say, "hold that thought, I need to focus until I get through this intersection," while waiting to turn left. My excuse was that I liked that little extra margin of driving safety.

Or my wife would say *this or that* was happening on the Internet, while I was trying to make coffee. I'd always respond back, "Hold that thought while I focus on getting this coffee made."

I'd constantly use the expression, "Hold that thought, while I focus on 'this or that'." All day long, every day of the week, for the past 18 months, at least, I began needing this more singular -concentrated focus on some activities about five years ago. This verbal communication behavior was very obvious to me and again, I just attributed it all to my neck being out of alignment and the aging process. After all, I was 63 years old.

Verbal Communication

My ability to think creatively and verbally communicate effectively began at a very early age. This ability was exercised and advanced all my life, until we moved to France. I've been selling or promoting something or other since I was 9 years old. Let me explain.

Dear Reader, you may be wondering where is this wandering Chapter 12 headed.

This chapter is my reality check. This chapter is like a breathalyzer sobriety test after drinking the Teasel Elixir for the past 23 days. This chapter is a review.

I asked in the beginning of this chapter with question number 2: A.m. I improving? Compared to what? Is my mental capability improving since I downed the first potent shot of Teasel Elixir? I need to know definitively.

This entire Chapter 12 review narrative is my roadside mental reality check on this personal journey. This is my chance to evaluate if I'm winning or losing on my verbal, cognitive and physical capacity over the past 23 days.

The Sales Profession

Selling may be one of the most maligned professions in the

world. That I think, because the term "selling" is very often confused with boorish manipulative skullthuggery, designed to twist hard earned dollars out of a person's wallet or purse with no respect or regard for the purse holder's natural self-interest. We humans have all been there for a fleecing, whether by a slippery-slimy-sleazy Sam, or a devious-diva Sally, or a do-gooder righteous religious Robert. Manipulative people are everywhere. Since the beginning of time.

Professional people, lay people, trades people, religious people, any kind of people can be manipulative, abusive, and on-the- make for our money, our time, or even our integrity and principle. That's not selling. That's theft.

Selling, to me, is the exchange of information about something that the "seller" is aware of, and that, the b*uyer*, may be interested in further exploring if . . . it's of interest to the buyer at that particular time and place. A salesperson's core attribute, core contribution in life, is to be a useful broker of good and useful information to any willing listener in need of such information.

To me, selling deals with individual things like a box of the suggested Lyme Protocol for 30 days. That's selling.

Promotion, to me, is the very same thing as selling, but with one key difference. Promotion, to me, is advancing the possibility of something big, something sweeping in scope, some big overarching idea, not a single box of vitamins.

Yes, Glidden is selling his individual protocol, but he's more so, steadfastly promoting naturopathic healing. He's both a salesman and a promoter, hand and glove, in my opinion. Dr. Glidden, Dr. Storl and Dr. Halverstadt all provided an information bridge from what they knew . . . to what I wanted to know: How to get rid of Lyme disease. That's what selling is all about: Information and idea exchanges through humanistic communication.

Promotion could be advocating that we keep the United States Constitutional Second Amendment intact so that we can all carry a Glock 9 automatic pistol down to the mall while shopping. Peddling a Glock 9 across the counter for eight hundred bucks isn't promotion, that's selling: Same arena of interest, but different scope of intention. One is big scale the other is small scale.

I use this hot issue only to accentuate the difference between selling and promotion. I'm ambivalent about things related to guns. I've hunted and shot a lot of things that I could roast over an open fire and eat. I've owned guns that were as beautiful as fine art work. Today I own none. I need none. Tomorrow I might own an arsenal but I pray not.

Today on this farm, I won't even kill a fly in the house. I just chase them out through an open window.

The effective sales person understands that it's up to the client, the listener, the prospect, or the courtroom jury for that matter, to, *Look, Listen and Decide.* The salesperson doesn't decide the outcome, the promoter doesn't determine the outcome . . . the client decides the outcome, without coercion or pressure. It was my job to, look, listen, and decide if I want to try these nutritional supplements and Storl's Teasel idea for healing.

Sales people and promoters alike who learn this philosophy and live this philosophy are some of the happiest and most career satisfied people on the planet, because they're truly helping people discover something of value, something they never knew about before or knew was possible before that salesperson entered their word. That's a very good feeling that no amount of money can buy. My entire life I've been selling something . . . and often not to earn money

Selling is a high-level verbal activity that requires focused concentration to be effective.

This is true for the Secretary of State for the United States selling a peace treaty between two warring nations or a clerk helping a new mother find a nice baby blanket for her first newborn child. Helping people is a wonderful thing. Selling, sharing information, or promoting a big idea can be the express route into that realm of helping people like no other profession. I've experienced that feelingly all my life. I like sharing good things with others.

My Communication Career Began Early

I started this phase of my life early, October, 1961, at age 9, and it stayed central and present in my life until it finally disappeared about two years ago, after my tool project and promotion ended with STIHL. That's about the time frame when my *Lyme-Lights* dimmed so low that helping others with good information or ideas sputtered to an end. "I was getting too old to help anyone anymore," I thought. This was the end of a long storied career that lasted over fifty years: Selling, promotion, and sharing inspiring ideas with others to make for a better world had finally come to an end for Jim.

I wanted a new bicycle that my parents weren't about to buy me. I wanted that bike, not to visit my friends, I wanted that bike to work on a strawberry farm just a few miles away, when I turned age twelve. I needed transportation to get to that job on the farm. That farm was going to gain me the financial freedom to hit the road permanently a few years down the line. It was all a dream until it came true.

I sold greeting cards door to door. That's how I began my lengthy communication career. In the back of a boys' magazine there was an ad offering all comers the opportunity to earn points toward receiving rewards in their merchandise catalogue. Therein was my bike. A beautiful Raleigh English 3-speed with saddlebags, hand brakes, a tire pump and plastic colored streamers. That was going to be my transportation up to the strawberry farm by the time I was twelve years old. It became a 2-year project selling house to country house, Thanksgiving, Christmas, and Easter cards, one or two boxes at a time, 25 cents profit per box, tax-free. That bike was earned on points because no cash ever flowed through a 9-year-old's hands. Cash wasn't that card company's system. I became an information broker at age 9 and learned some wonderful lessons that stayed with me a lifetime. I'm forever grateful how that stroke of fate shaped my entire life. Let me explain.

My First Sale

My first sale was to a neighbor lady, a farmer's wife. They owned a beautiful small apple orchard across the road. It was to her that my first sales pitch just flowed out of my mouth with absolutely no forethought. I suspect the radio receiver was turned on and somebody was helping me out again because a 9-year-old doesn't come up with a simple sale pitch . . . but I did that day, and here is how I got that Raleigh bike. Almost word for word, I remember my presentation from 54 years ago like yesterday.

Me: I knock on the door.

Home Owner: Opens the door.

Me: "Hello, I'm here to offer special greeting cards for Thanksgiving, Christmas and Easter. They're special and different because they can be customized with your own personal message. They cost no more because there's no middleman but me, and they're delivered direct to your home by the company."

I stopped there for any kind of response. But usually got invited inside.

Once inside I continued: "Can I show you what they look like?"

With the sales book open, the focus was on them deciding what they liked among 100's and 100's of beautiful cards for all tastes. Boxed in either 25 or 50, no mixing. At that stage, they couldn't say no, no matter what month it was because there was always one of the three holidays on the horizon. I sold October to Easter for two years. The 2nd year it was mostly all repeat business. I just knocked on the same doors to see if there was a new message, i.e., newborns to add etc.

Once they decided what they wanted, I handed them the form to fill out for all their shipping information and their custom message, in their handwriting, not mine.

When it got to payment details, I explained that I was too young to handle any money and that this company only took checks paid directly to the card company. I told them I was paid with points, not cash.

That comment usually sparked a bit of curiosity about my motivation for this sales activity. From that point on I always made sure to work the following magic kryptonite into the conversation.

Me: I'd pull out the treasure catalogue with that Raleigh three speed Bike equipped with basket and streamers and point to it with pride and say: "You'll receive the cards in a few weeks, and I'll receive some points for this bike, which will become my transportation in two years up to the strawberry farm for work when I'm 12 years old."

Everybody knew about this iconic second generation Strawberry farm, if was the biggest one in a 500-mile radius.

Out the door, I walked from that apple orchard, down their country driveway to the next house however far away it was. I walked those country roads for two seasons, October to April, a lot of it in snow and rain after school and on weekends until I had my bike in the Spring of 1963. When I was 11 years old with my own bike, it became a gateway to the entire world.

Two Wealthy Sisters

With my first sale in hand, I walked the other direction down the busy highway toward the biggest mansion in the county . . . at least I thought it was the biggest. Most of the housing stock we all lived in, back then, would be considered teardown specials today. Small bungalows, and tiny old drafty craftsmen farm houses, most with full running water and plumbing, some partially without. Tiny homes by today's standards, all occupied by depression era parents who were struggling after WWII to build their families, us baby boomers. I was just one more kid in that rural scrambled community mix.

These ladies that I was going to see were wealthy. It was rumored that these two elderly sisters made their fortune designing spelling books for grade school children. Their spelling books made them their fortune and they built a beautiful estate, which to me at age 9 looked like *Tara* in *Gone With The Wind*. That was my impression. That was my next stop for an introduction of my cards. Neither I, nor anybody in the entire county that I knew about, had ever been inside their mansion. These sisters were people that our community gossiped about but rarely saw in public. It was a hidden mansion backed deep into their wooded property connected by a long curved gravel driveway out to the paved main highway.

I noticed the driveway gravel texture immediately when walking up to their house. I had never felt anything underfoot quite like it before and not again until forty years later did I experience that same quiet soft feel underfoot until walking the courtyards of the Queen's Buckingham Palace in London. It was gravel meant for fancy horses and carriages to tread upon. Their long winding driveway was quiet, soft and uniform to walk upon, a special gravel, not like the chunky sharp stuff laid down in everybody else's driveway. I felt right then and there that this was a special place, even if everybody gossiped about these two older sisters who lived there.

I was ready for my second sale, it was an afternoon in October, when a 9-year-old kid knocked on the door, and it swung open. The owner I presumed, an old lady, elegant, a tall figure who stood her ground in the middle of the doorframe silently and just stared at me.

A *man's* voice from around the corner and out of sight from me, a very unusual voice, said, "Hello." The lady just stood and stared at me. The deep voice repeated again, "Hello."

The lady threw me a huge friendly smile and said come on in, walked me around the blind corner and introduced me to her friend, a beautiful talking bird in a cage at least ten feet tall. That drawing room was like nothing I had ever seen. It was a majestic brick and wood mansion full of light and beauty. That was my impression and still is to this very day . . . a house full of bright natural light. Later I'd eventually learn much more about these remarkable aging sisters.

I went through the presentation, she ordered some cards, and we became friends. I revisited her mansion many times before I began working on the strawberry farm and remember her fondly. I never did meet her sister. People gossiped that these two lady spinsters were unusual, but to me, she was this wonderful beautiful soul, living quietly back in the forest with her sister, creating school books for children across America, was like some type of spiritual Angel.

From that day forward I felt like the hand of God himself was clearing a path for me and that nice lady must have been my appointed patron saint. I'm not sure if she didn't call everybody in the county to tell them if they didn't buy the cards, she would do it for them. I don't ever remember customers turning me down. It was an incredible feeling to be welcomed into stranger's homes wherever I walked in, offering them nice pretty cards to brighten up their life.

From that time forward, I took up every opportunity to communicate publicly. It was like I had started a fire at 9 years old, and I just kept throwing more logs onto the heap as my experience burned brighter and brighter with every selling and speaking experience for the next fifty years.

Early Lessons In Basic Human Diplomacy

After the first two seasons on the strawberry farm, by age 14, I became an accomplished field boss during picking season, expert at parking hundreds and hundreds of cars, rain or shine, seven days per week, then herding these car people across fields of fresh ripe strawberries and keeping them all peaceful, right out to the finish line at the cashiers stand. These berry fields were a public speaking experience extraordinaire. It was dynamic and serious if not fun because it involved masses and mobs of interesting people who all wanted something *right now!* Fresh morning strawberries. Let me explain.

This was a unique pick-your-own operation and it was on this farm I leaned diplomacy and leadership at an almost spiritual level. At 7:00 a.m. for three weeks in June and July, upwards of a thousand plus anxious people were ready to rush into the fields to attack the berry patch. It had to be kept orderly, neat, and tidy for the next day's picking or it would've tuned into a giant muddy mess with destruction and chaos from stem to stern. Strawberries ripen very fast and rot very quickly in late June and July heat. They all have to be picked on time or the whole field can rot out very quickly.

It was a mad scramble for three hectic weeks. Thousands upon thousands of city people, mostly older family women, sometimes with their children and grandparents and dogs. Many were Polish or Italian immigrants with limited English capability.

Four or five field bosses would shepherd and guide this swarming mass with few words, combined with police like hand signals, to direct the human flow: "You go here, you stay there, the potty place is over there in the woods, we don't supply toilet paper, control your dog, control your children, pick all the red ones, don't squash down your neighbor's row."

We were like human sheep dogs steering the flock were to graze. It was a sight to behold and it seemed to work beautifully. Many of these big city people had never set foot on farm dirt before and it was like a wonderful cultural exchange for everybody, including me.

It was wild and crazy for about four to five hours each morning until the sun got too hot, or the berries ran out, or the pickers had enough country living for one day. They would pay the cashiers when they had their fill and drive away. Later we usually fired up the irrigation system to water everything down nice and cool, ripening those berries for the next day to start all over again.

Pick your own strawberries is a very lucrative cash crop if a farmer gets everything just right. Most never do, but this operation worked like magic. The key was to get the berries to peak perfection one day, and pick them the next. If they weren't picked almost immediately, they rotted into bird food and spoiled every berry they touched like a fast burning fire. It's very difficult to run a successful pick you own berry patch, but this farm, is still running like a top today after almost 80 years in its fifth generation of family ownership. Their family name is legendary in the strawberry business worldwide, because that owner I worked for traveled the world to freely share his secrets of strawberry success. They made it look easy. It's not. I did that for five summers and it's where I learned many things, but it was the verbal communication and the human diplomacy that I learned, far beyond my years, that I remember most.

I loved that farm. Many young men had gone before me, and many after. That's why it was a prize to get a job there. Young men talked about that farm as a temporary life destination and not a job. The owner was a family man of unique disposition and patient humanitarian wisdom. His operation to us young men was a cross hybrid experience like a paid summer camp mixed together with a heavy side order of commercial agribusiness. We operated, we fixed and we repaired everything: tractors and transmissions and trucks and hay balers, pumps, engines, bearings and brakes, shotguns and firecrackers for bird control, sprayers, herbicides, pesticides, plows, harrows, welders and grinders, cutting torches and fabricating jigs, painting and patching, tire repairs and trips to the railhead with trucks and trailers driven down the public highways by me . . . underage . . . with farm license legality.

Post picking season during late summer break, we had barbeques and canoe camping trips with the owner, and many hours down at the irrigation-swimming hole. This all transpired for me between the ages of 12 to 17. It was amazing. I had no interest in summer baseball or anything related to sports. I lived in a *paradise lost* on that farm and my bicycle got me to paradise each day.

It was like a paid 3-month summer scholarship to the *Ivy League* of real life. Leadership, communication, and responsibility, which I learned there, have stayed with me for a lifetime. That work experience at such an early age, I believe, is unprecedented how us young men leaned to communicate and get along with people of wide diversity and temperament.

This was a step up from selling cards door to door. I'll never forget that very first paycheck I clutched in my hand June of 1964 at age 12, flying downhill from the farm on payday towards home, free as a bird on that day with streamers flying out horizontal in the slipstream. I was the happiest kid in the world because my escape plan was intact to leave one day from a miserable household of domestic toxicity brought on by a deeply troubled husband mired in a lifetime of self-centered loveless misery.

Towards A Grand Final Review

I completely understand if you're lost with boredom by now, and are asking yourself when all this pointless trivia is going to end. I can assure you these past 20 pages aren't for your benefit, although some of the words might be interesting to a young boy, who'll read these tales of old like a dusty old Hardy Boys Book from an irrelevant era, long past and forgotten.

No, Dear Reader, theses past 20 pages are for me. I'm in a deeply introspective process of asking and will eventually need to answer that very basic second question I posed to myself 5,745 words ago: Is my brain along with my body, my spirit and my emotions getting any better since I began this Teasel program a bit over three weeks ago, or am I wasting my time and money deluding myself . . . and further more . . . compared to what? That's the question for me . . . "compared to what?" How am I doing today compared to yesterday, last week, and last year, compared to the last five decades?

Every last thought put to paper in this chapter came to me in a flash, like a life review when a person is dying. In an instant these mini movies of early adolescent life and a whole lot more rolled thought my mind when I asked myself how are my basic cognitive facilities doing? Am I winning or am I losing ground, and if so, how good or how bad? I need comparative data to know and the only thing I can compare is all of my life experiences. I can't measure cognitive ability and motivation levels like a runner on a racetrack with a stopwatch or a sweating groaning gym rat on an exercise machine. I want to know how is my brain functioning. Only I can answer that question as I sit isolated on our farm in old rural France reviewing these mental mini flashes. They're being written down here for review and comparison, to be rolled over and over and pondered for months and years into the future. Am I better off mentally now than yesterday and compared to what?

Yes, I can measure distance walked and pounds lifted, that's easy, but I'm not trying to measure those physical things. That's what the 500-meter field circuit around the farm fence line is for, and I know for sure, I do have a very long way to go before I'll ever be chasing that badminton birdie . . . if ever.

However, If the chiropractors and healers are right, and the worst does get fixed first, I suspect it was my mind and my brain that were in far worse shape than my knee. I can see that clearly now. My knee, if it ever grows some cartilage back, is far less important than getting my attitude, and state of depression and cognitive abilities back on track and healthy and fully functioning again. I believe that's happening very quickly in some almost mysterious ways.

This life review continues for one more mini movie: The Catholic Church.

Oratory From The Pulpit

This passage about the Pulpit will be my last element in review from the past. I know it's time to move on, because I can see the end of this book in sight, and where it's all heading in a few months' time: Picnics. Yes that's right . . . Picnics. The recent incoming bolts, like those transmissions I received on that ridge top in Laguna, tells me there are lots of summer picnics coming. Picnics and what they mean will be the final chapter of this book in a few months to come. This metaphoric concept, grounded in reality, and now indelibly printed in my thinking, will never be lost, but it'll have to wait for later because I have some serious healing that needs attending to before that last chapter on picnics.

The Church

As much as I loved that strawberry farm and working there 700 hours each summer, I loved even more the nine months I spent each year in Catholic school from grade four through grade eight. If that farm was a *paradise lost*, that Catholic Grade School was *heaven on earth*.

Formal education wasn't always that way for me before or after those five glorious Catholic School years. My Catholic School education for the first three grades before *heaven on earth* was located in the *Devil's Paradise of Hell*. When I entered Hell, that first religious-sponsored catastrophe for half-day Kindergarten class, I began stalling out on three spoken words: My last name, "Lindl", the article word, "a" and the color word "yellow".

Those three words were roadblocks that caused my speech to go full stop. I had others, but these three were the biggest troublemakers particularly the "a" and the "yellow". The last name was an easy one for me because I just avoided being a Lindl. It was the article "a" that came out like full-auto rips from an unbridled AK47 Kalashnikov rifle. It was always the soft "a" as in cat, or hat, or tap. Those soft "a" words were an absolute impossibility to pronounce without going full auto Kalashnikov.

The "yellows" never even crossed my lips, they just stopped dead, down deep inside, somewhere far deeper than any psychologist could ever determine. Even just the thought of "yellow" never traveled past my solar plexus where it caused everything to shut down full stop in self-conscious fear of ridicule. "Yellow" was the baddie for me, full of deep shame to pronounce. Sometimes the Kalashnikov "Kah, ah, ah . . . ah, ah, ah, ah . . . ah, ah, ah, ah, aht", garnered compassion, but the "yellow" stall-out reflex usually precipitated puzzlement or ridicule or irritation and laughter by the listeners of a 7-year-old boy in Catholic Grade school. Those Nuns, and sometimes a few children, would stare at my shameful silence accompanied by their derisory cackles and clucking.

By the end of 3rd grade, I can't tell you how many times I stood in the corner for punishment, or peed my pants in class because I stalled out, locked up and couldn't talk. The nuns thought I was being an obstinate disobedient little shit, unknown to them that I was stuck on the "yellow".

Today I feel sorry for the misery that must have swirled around those nuns to become so cruel to so many young children. I'm not sorry for the Nuns. I'm sorry for the misery that swirled throughout their realm that must have infected so many young people. There's a difference . . . those Nuns were adults and I'm not sorry for them, I'm sorry for the toxicity of their world . . . they had a choice to do the right thing or walk out and quite. We all have the choice . . . to do the right thing . . . if we so chose, but often it's the most difficult thing in our lives to act upon principle rather than life expediency.

Those painful experiences built strength in me, and resolve like kryptonite steel . . . not anger or resentment, but resolve against injustice. It built resolve to never be hurt. Military people in the know told me later in life that I would've made a good Special Forces covert operative because of the emotional distance I could create around my exterior shell. That ability to create emotional separation is what allowed us timber cutters to disengage from the constant fear that could grip a person while performing the most lethal work on planet earth.

Thankfully, I walked out of that grade school intact unlike those thousands of Native Indian Kids buried behind the Catholic Orphanage schools and their dormitories scattered across Northern Canada on the fringes of civilization.

Everything eventually got all nicely turned around in the next school of bright energetic and happy singing nuns who treated us with love and respect. The stuttering persisted well into adulthood but like every stutterer, I eventually learned in my own way how to cover this embarrassing impediment. My cover was learned from the Church Pulpit . . . the dramatic orator's pause or the look away glance from the listener. These speech devices became my stuttering bridge among the tough words that wouldn't flow out easily into the fluid stream of normal speech.

My father had the same affliction with "Lindl" and never attempted to get it out. I remember to this day very clearly how on the phone, on in person, he would bridge past his first name while always skipping his last name during self-introduction for personal identity. I never heard him utter his last name once in the 17 years I lived in that household. He must've never got the memo on the orator's pause.

The Orator's Pause

Here is how I define the orator's pause: The orator's pause isn't some contrived art form of public speaking. In fact, true oratory can't be contrived at all because it comes deep from within the speaker's heart. It's a brief naturally timed bridge between deeply held beliefs, often of a passionate nature.

The orator's or speaker's pause, is that sublime moment between two thoughts, certainly much longer that a comma, but also longer than even the mental breathing space provided by a period.

The orator's pause is an indication to the listener that something profound has just been spoken, or that something is about to be announced in the next breath implying . . . some very important thought is on its way.

No doubt you've noticed my extensive use of . . . followed by another thought. These three dots are put in to suggest that what *was* written or is *about* to be written is weighty enough to pause and ponder.

The orator's pause is a respectful mental interlude that the orator realizes the listener needs to fully absorb and metabolize a spoken phrase before moving on to the next piece of thinking being conveyed to the listener.

Sincere Oratory isn't a contrivance because it comes from the heart . . . not from a teleprompter.

Did you feel that 3-dot pause before, *"not from a Teleprompter?"* I wanted to make a point that today's politicians aren't like John F. Kennedy, or Martin Luther King Jr., or Sir Winston Churchill, or Abraham Lincoln. These historical statesmen had passion and belief behind their message. Could you imagine Martin Luther King Jr. reading off a Teleprompter? Not in a million years. Dr. King wasn't looking to score a few sound bite points from a teleprompter-like canned speech in the next opinion polls. He was looking to change the broad sweep history . . . and he did.

Doctor Martin Luther King Jr. was probably the most passionate orator of our age, a man so gifted with his message that he moved an entire nation with his love and truth . . . all with his oratory. That's why he was feared. He was murdered because he had love in his heart and didn't need guns to change the world . . . only words from his heart. His heart is what petrified the people who had no love in their heart and only knew how to control and rule their agenda with their self-serving laws, dictates and guns.

Same with Kennedy and Gandhi and others throughout history. Their hearts were too powerful to contain so they were assassinated. That's the power of passionate oratory.

Here is Dr. King's written opening in his, *I have a dream speech*:

"I am happy to join with you today . . . in what will go down in history . . . as the greatest demonstration for freedom in the history of our Nation."

Notice the three dot pauses, which you can listen to on the audio below.

Linked below is his live speech from August 28th, 1963. Please listen for the oratory pauses that allow the listener to metabolize his breathtaking bold message of . . . *I have a Dream*. Dear Reader, this speech's finale can bring the dead back to life if ever that was possible by a human being. I wonder how many grade school kids or high school kids today ever heard this speech of such pivotal history shaping importance. Martin Luther King, Jr. - I Have A Dream (from American Rhetoric)

I became an orator in Church by necessity. Latin, embroidered satin cassocks and ringing bells weren't my cup of tea so altar boy duties were out of the question. I was a country kid who wore blue jeans and work boots with ground-in grease on my calloused hands and tractor blood in my veins. I wasn't material for the obligatory altar boy rotational call-out for every grade school male in that wonderful school I called heaven. Those Nuns could read my situation so they gave me pulpit duty five mornings each week at the before school compulsory school kids' Mass.

Rarely was anybody in there but a couple of Nuns and all

the kids who weren't dragging their feet to school. Sometimes when the weather was cold a drunk or two sat in the back, but we pretty much had the place to ourselves every morning until the mass ended at 9:00 a.m.

My job was to hop up to the Pulpit at the appropriate time and read a bit of the liturgy and the daily bulletins if anything new was happening.

I did that for almost five years and I had to overcome my stuttering. Although "Lindl" and "yellow" never came into the mix there were plenty of soft "a's" that were just waiting to turn into a bust of stuttering gunfire across the pews.

I certainly knew nothing about the orator's gentle pause . . . nor did the church organist, but she knew how to control her own stuttering by simply pausing for a moment before the tough words that might cause some troubles. It was through her gentle kind coaching and the kindness of all the nuns and my classmates, that I transitioned from a quaking peeing insecure mess, to class President. I was asked to give the commencement speech at the end of eighth grade final graduation in 1966 in the school gymnasium with all the Nuns and 7th graders, along with their families in attendance. It was a glorious event for everybody, which included a nice big lunch and festivities. This school was heaven on earth to me and I was surrounded by my wonderful happy fiends and all their proud parents.

I was introduced by the head priest to the graduating assembly by first and last name so I had that covered . . . the rest went really well because I made sure to include no "yellows" into the speech. Unfortunately, for my father that day . . . he missed his chance to see his son use the oratory pause. He missed his chance for a stuttering lesson from his own son, because he didn't have the time to attend that glorious grade eight final graduation. He did have time for his lake front cabin that he had officially named *The Alibi*, doing some sort of weekend work project. If nothing else, I found him to always to be a transparent and truthful man. I never knew him to lie to anybody with his words . . . but most importantly . . . his actions. May his soul rest in peace.

The Final Review

Saturday, January 2, 2016, 4:49 a.m.

Dear Reader, it has taken me 6 days, 8,629 words and 29 pages of keystrokes to arrive at all these Chapter 12 concluding remarks 28 days after beginning this holistic healing protocol.

Interesting, to me, how fast the brain can process a few simple thoughts in an instant, but the written or verbal expression of those thoughts can lag so far behind. That's one of the inherent malfunctions of stuttering and ADD/ADHD. The brain is far ahead of the mouth, and the two are simply not synchronized. Mix in some fear into the mess and presto, the stuttering begins firing full-auto until the cycle of stuttering is broken by some intervening catalyst like a smack from a Catholic Nun, or the orators pause.

Everything, well almost everything, in these entire preceding 29 pages flashed through my mind in an instant when I asked the question seven days ago:

Am I improving? . . . Compared to What?

When I asked that question seven days ago, I immediately knew the answer. Let me explain.

There's no question my knee is better today, four weeks to the day that I began the Teasel and this high powered nutritional support. I'm thankful and hopeful at the same time. Thankful for what knee improvement I have today and hopeful there's more and better to come. God willing, I'll be chasing that birdie by June, but it has a long way to go.

On The Physical, Muscular & Structural Side

The hot knee syndrome never returned after beginning the fish oil pills on the second day. I can definitely walk the 500-meter circuit and probably much more if I chose, but I try to minimize any walking because I'm trying to re-grow the cartilage and I fear that excessive unnecessary joint movement will just grind down anything that may be starting to come back.

My knee isn't sharply painful like the months before taking all these vitamins, but it'll still get quite uncomfortable after walking and it's definitely telling me to be careful. If I was in Paris, would I walk that city mile down concrete sidewalks to get a Starbucks coffee today? Not in a million years. That would be just plain foolish behavior at this juncture of healing. I feel that it'll be months before that bone on bone conditions will improve, but to me, that's a lot quicker and better than struggling though a dangerous 12-month rehab the Périgueux surgeon promised was in the cards if I go under the knife. I plan on getting an x-ray taken at the 3rd and the 6th month marker to check for cartilage growth: First week of March and first week of June X-rays don't lie.

The only thing I'll be doing differently in addition to the specified products for my knee cartilage is drinking some Horsetail Herbal Tea twice daily for Cartilage regeneration. The balance of the protocol will remain for the next 60 days and the subject of Horsetail Plants is the topic for the next chapter. I began drinking this tea two days ago after my wife alerted me to the benefits of this tea while reading Matthew

Wood's seminal writing on herbal healing in *The Book of Herbal Wisdom*. Horsetail herbal therapy is supposed to be the miracle herb for cartilage repair like Tease magic is for Lyme disease. Interesting to me is that we have wild horsetail growing along our river frontage. That's two for two in our neighborhood: Wild Teasel growing 250 meters from our house and the feathery soft Horsetail herb plant about 75 meters downstream from this very keyboard. My holistic solutions are once again . . . hiding in plain sight. The Book Of Herbal Wisdom, by Matthew Wood (woodherbs.com)

On The Respiratory Side

I haven't written much about my respiratory system these past 28 days. There's also some nice improvement. Remarkable improvement actually.

Aware mountain guides introducing novice climbers to the alpine world, especially those short trips where the climbers pop up over 12,000 foot elevation quickly from sea level, have to pay extra close attention to their parties breathing to keep everybody safe. One of the easiest indicators of safety and climber stability is the ability of all in the group to continue talking while climbing. When inexperienced climbers launch out of Lake Helen their jocular banter may be prevalent, but any cockiness diminishes quickly as basic conversation in the thin air becomes difficult. If the climbers are overstressing their respiratory system, the talking stops.

That's the indicator of an overstressed vertical ascent and the pace needs to be slowed down. Verbal communication goes down first with oxygen deprivation. If they keep climbing too fast and the talking never resumes, between 12,500 and 13,500, the dry heaves and vomiting can begin and they usually turn back down with massive headaches. For some, it can become deadly dangerous to be running down their oxygen level that rapidly and their blood gasses get so far out of whack they can't recover and they die. It happens on Shasta and other popular climbs where novices think an alpine climb from 7,000 to 14,000-foot elevation is some weekend walk in the park. Altitude Sickness (Altitude.org)

I'm acutely aware of my breathing state. I don't smoke. I drink some red wine and occasional Champaign, but only in moderation. My resting pulse rate at bed rise is in the low 50's and runs mid 60's during the day unless I kick into some physical activity.

Beginning about a year ago, I could feel shortness of breath after walking up the very slight hill to our mailbox. No more than 25 feet of elevation gain over 160 meters of length. That got my attention but it only got worse. Twenty-eight days ago before starting the full protocol, when climbing up one flight of steps to my wife's office in our home, I had to take in a few shallow breaths before talking when I arrived on the second floor. It was like I had just cleared 12,500 feet punching upward a bit too fast to the top of Shasta with a 25-pound pack. That was my breathing state 28 days ago. I couldn't walk up one flight of steps without running short of breath. My wife noticed this very obvious condition as well. This isn't the Jim Lindl, firewood splitting, fence pounding farmer and mountaineer, she knew from a few years ago.

Today, 28 days into the Teasel and the nutritional regime and I can stand beside a pile of tough round wood, and wail away at a it with a 2.6 kilo blunt edge spitting mall and work till I'm drenched in sweat without getting short of breath. The mailbox hill and steps are now easy to climb with no apparent diminishment of respiratory capacity during any of my day-to-day activity. This past week I've used the Lawn tractor very little to get around our little farm unless there's something to carry. Three months ago, I never walked to the mailbox and back because of the knee pain and the short breathing. I do that easily today, four weeks into this holistic cure. I'm thankful.

Only by climbing vigorously with a mountain pack or spinning a mountain bike up through our rolling hill country could I determine the maximum level of my breathing efficiency, but for now, my right knee won't allow that much joint pressure. However, I can report that my breathing is better now than it has been for several years. I believe that the Lyme bacteria must have been attacking just about my entire body and shutting everything down pretty tightly to the point of basic survival just 28 days ago. I'm very thankful that I can breathe normally again.

On The Pulmonary Side

I'm pleased to report that none of the heart racing and erratic blood pressure spikes I experience August, September, October and November have recurred in the past 28 days.

My first surprise blood pressure reading occurred in Dr. Halverstadt's office in California. I was surprised and asked for a retake on the opposite arm. It was confirmed that I had uncomfortably high blood pressure. It's probably recorded in his notes but I do remember it running in the mid 150's over low 90's on both arms. That shocked me because I've never had any history of unusual blood pressure or a high resting pulse rate. I continued to check these vitals up to December 5th where the pressure ran erratically between my normal 120's over 60's/low 80's. to the high Halverstadt levels. Bizarre how the blood pressure could spike up and then settle down in a 24-hour period without any provocation or dietary change.

Saturday, January 02, 2016, 9:57 p.m.

It's now two hours since a big diner and a nice glass of red wine. I just left the keyboard, bounced up the stairs to the second floor and checked my blood pressure for this report. It clocked in at 127/70 with a pulse rate of 77 per minute. Given that I had a glass of wine, and it's pretty hot beside the fire right now, I think that's a pretty respectable end of day blood pressure and pulse reading. That reading range has been the norm for the past couple of weeks but with a resting pulse in the 60's. Before this healing process began December 5th, my blood pressure was erratic all day long. I believe the Lyme bacteria are once again responsible for these past blood pressure issues.

Since my August scare with spontaneous unprovoked runaway heart racing, upwards of 200 beats per minute, I've had no further serious episodes. That racing heart condition is what scared me into calling the California guitar picking Chiropractor who gifted me Egoscue's book. Ironically, I'm thankful for those heart palpitating attacks, because without them, I may have never gone to California and had that fortuitous meeting with Dr. Halverstadt, who started me looking into Lyme bacteria as a potential root cause of all these obvious systemic malfunctions. Everything seems to happen for a reason so long as we keep our eyes peeled.

The Grand Finale Of Changes In The Past 30 Days

Sunday, January 03, 2016, 4:09 a.m.

On The Verbal, Cognitive & Motivational Side

The changes have been absolutely stunning . . . beyond my wildest expectations. . . all very positive.

No doubt, you've noted a few behavioral changes, maybe some attitude shifts, certain mental peculiarities about this writer over the past four weeks who is now pounding more keystrokes at 4:00 a.m. This early bird rise might suggest he's not even close to his mental grave.

With this writer's off the wall passages about dog farts and a canine's interpretation of a master's vulgarity, mixed with comments about a cesium clock's role in GPS signal calibration, juxtaposed to American Monetary theory received from outer space . . . if not total delirium . . . at least his writing indicates robust activity in his verbal and cognitive process.

I'm not going crazy. Rather I'm more like a young boy who has been let out of bondage after being cooped up in the orphanage of his slowly dying mind for the past seven years, and am now running around the outdoor mental playground of life, like the happiest and freest kid in the world. That's about how my brain feels after being on the Teasel tincture for 29 days.

CK is a trusted Montana friend and my supplier for all these products.

I've been on the phone with CK weekly since she discovered for me that naturopathic video lecture series floating out in the star field, far outside my shortsighted and biased tunnel vision.

She and I have exceptional history that goes back over 20 years to the beginning of our startup vitamin business in 1993. She's been the key to organizing all my product deliveries from California to France, as well as a trusted sounding board in the healing process over the past month. She doesn't think I've gone nuts, which is reassuring.

She just thinks I've turned into a chatter box on the phone, like a young excited kid, whose brain got recently turned back on . . . back to the old Jim Lindl she knew 23 years ago when we started up our company with two venture capitalists and a hand full of other excited dedicated believers. She's noticed in me, over these past four weeks, a total 360° transformation big time, beginning about one week after starting this powerful nutritional healing regime and the mysterious Teasel herbal concoction. Her valued feedback is a welcome realistic benchmark of my continuing cognitive mental recovery.

Long Conversations At Home

I believe we can do anything we want to in life, just not all at the same time, or we'll probably make a mess of the whole lot. Success takes focused concentration for the period of time a specific task requires. I know this immutable law of time management well, because I've lived it all my life. Whether selling greeting cards to buy a 3-speed Raleigh bike by age 12, or building a national vitamin empire in four years, the time management principles are always the same. Focused concentration is one of the master keys to getting projects done.

When a group of us built up our vitamin company, many of us had incredible laser-focus for several years. Myself particularly so, because I was tasked to build the entire distribution operation across 50 states, from scratch, which eventually mushroomed into 15,000 independent distributors by March 17, 1997, four years into the burn. It grew faster and bigger than everybody's expectations by miles. By that 48-month marker, I had a lot of free cash flowing my way, but also an equal if not more amount of free time flowing my way.

One of the things my wife and I did with some of that money and time was build a very nice house, which had gorgeous library floor-to-ceiling double hung wood sash windows in classic 1920's craftsman style.

In this very special airy bright room, she and I would sit each morning for a couple of leisurely hours and simply talk. We talked about a lot of different subjects back then: People, and places, ideas, dreams, and sorrows, money, religion, and politics, just life stuff . . . Maslow, and Freud, and Schatzman . . . Rothbard, Rand and Bastiat and justice for all . . . not just the privileged class. We would talk about timber cutting and gardening and coyotes and wild turkeys, rattlesnakes, skunks and our pet dog. We would just talk. It was a special room, in a very special house, during a very special period in our lives. We were young, we had earned some good money and we had earned some free time. We lived a simple good life for two people who both left home early, never inherited a nickel, never asked for more than was honestly earned and always paid our debts and taxes in full. That was our life back then.

Over time, those long conversations disappeared along with that house. Those conversions simply dried up like flowers in the sun. Then as my failing health took over these past seven years, even the thought of lingering conversation time like the old days, died for good. Recent short conversations in my state of fuzzy health centered on advancing age, failing health, month-to-month survival, health insurance, taxes, money, food, the weather, the dog. Pretty basic stuff and not much more. I couldn't and didn't think beyond the next month. I was in survival mode. Those days of old, with the daily conversation furnace burning brightly, were stone cold dead without even a tiny pilot light to ignite any free leisurely thinking. I didn't equate any of this to the maladies of the dreaded Lyme Spirochetes until reading Storl. He writes about the very spirit of life itself getting sucked out by Lyme disease.

That all got changed after a dozen days of Teasel shots before breakfast followed by two more stiff ones later in the day. After the bull bellowing and lion roaring spasms, the hot showers, and the mud pies, everything began to reignite in my verbal system and my brain began to come alive from the deeps.

My conversation brain gradually woke back up like *Rip Van Winkle* coming out of some deep fuzzy mental drift. I can't ever remember being this lucid and verbal as I sit at the computer today, but I sure will take what I have today for age 63. I hope this isn't one big temporary respite from the deep like *Awakenings*. Who knows. Time will tell. Awakenings (Wikipedia)

Most days now, for an hour or so, we sit by the fireplace, right beside this keyboard and talk. The dog lies there but doesn't care if we talk about healing herbs, Storl, Wood or Teasel . . . refugee camps, Putin or wars, or high taxes and other mundane things . . . just so long as we scratch his ears and let him know he's always our friend. He never asks for more, and could care less about all the rest of the world out there. No doubt, my cognitive and verbal communication ability is coming back stronger than ever. I'm thankful.

I'm thankful to be able to think, ponder, and communicate again. That began after the Teasel began to go down the hatch each morning, whose main job I thought, was to go kill off some nasty spirochetes. I didn't recognize how far I had slipped under the waves of solitude and depression until re-reading these pages of personal review and reflection. Storl does talk about these things related to Lyme disease, and now I know, firsthand, what he and others have experienced with this insidious Lyme toxicity that penetrates beyond the mind to one's very soul. I had become like the living dead.

I offer this Internet link below which describes the robust life of my past that had just slipped under the waves and was gone. This *LinkedIn* profile outlines my previous active farm life and previous Vitamin business, and an outline of other activities over the years: Gardening, Tool Invention, volunteer work and constructing that special house with the magic floor-to-ceiling bright airy windows. That was my past life and I thought everything was over, done and gone for good at my age of 63. I now have stirring motivation to add more to that profile in the future. I know that as I tap out these keystrokes . . . I'm back and alive with more than just a sputter of hope. Jim Lindl - LinkedIn

I definitely haven't felt this type of drive and motivation in many, many years. It all has come back since I began taking the Teasel. I'm thankful for my newfound motivation to live and be active again. My knee better hurry along to catch up with my brain though, because I have an appointment with the future. *"Worst first. Top down, Inside out."* I sincerely pray that's the healing sequence going on. If true, then my maligned knee joint can't be far behind.

Emotional Cleansing

On The Emotional Side

The recent change I've experienced has been very specific and singular in nature, but I believe hugely transformative, and as important as the other changes in this review chapter all combined together. Let me explain.

It's possible that people may think it's not very becoming for a rough-cut timber cutter to admit to some personal emotional issues. "Not very manly," they may think. Better left to not talk about these sensitive private things. Well, let me assure you, we loggers don't wear panty hose under our bulletproof Kevlar work chaps, yet are very comfortable exposing our private issues for the whole world to see in public without a second thought. If not always dignified, we loggers can be colorful and entertaining to watch in our times of emotional release.

What do you think knurly wood-whacking beasts are up to every time we let fly vulgar puss and spittle in our little boy fits of anger? Those episodes are nothing more than an abbreviated emotional cleansing in verbal form. Loggers do it all the time, probably every day about something. Sometimes these releases are nonverbal, entirely internal, like explosive mental steam released with the intensity of a drunken barroom brawl. Yes, we loggers have our ways to show the world when we have issues and aren't happy.

I think all people have emotional sensitivities and issues that need to be dealt with from time to time . . . or those issues will deal unkindly with us in return. Someone who never gets outwardly angry may be the angriest person in the neighborhood.

This singular and powerful emotional cleanse I experienced just recently, was entirely internal with no external expression. Nobody would've ever known what happened

Let me explain.

My Big Surprise

I don't get surprised very often in life. My wife and I haven't lived exactly a plain vanilla life, but we definitely try to organize and structure our day-to-day life to minimize anything resembling a surprise.

September of 1990, I was sitting at our home office desk while the wife and I were ready to launch out the door to Cabo San Lucas for some sun. We were almost ready to leave when the phone rang. I picked it up and it was a surprise like none other in my life.

It was my father! WOW!! Nothing changed since I left home at age 17, he still couldn't pronounce his last name. Addressing me as his son or as my father was equally out of the question. He used his old phone bridge technique to get past his last name and got on with the conversation.

This was a major surprise out of the blue because this was the *first time* and the *only time* until he died in his eighties that he ever picked up the phone to call me. That's exactly right. My very earliest childhood recollections up to the day I left home at age 17, is that he had neither the time nor the desire to converse with me unless for some absolute irritating necessity, and that emotional distance remained up to the day he died. That's how I remember him to this day and that indelible perception has remained my reality for 63 years: I was the time wasting irrelevant son in his life.

From the day I left home at age 17, I had no desire to talk to him either. I was an irrelevant, if not irritating inconvenience to him for the first 17 years of my life, and he became equally irrelevant to me for the remainder of my life. Apparently, however, this day was a special occasion for him to call unannounced after 21 years of me leaving home. So I asked, "What's up?" in a tone like I'm talking to the meter-reader out at the power pole checking the home's power consumption. Keeping this special father-son relationship in perspective, I found it quite normal that our very brief conversation lasted at most . . . two minutes. The first time he called me in my life when I'm 38 years old.

Of course, he didn't ask how was the wife, or me, or life, or my health, or the dog, or the dog's health, or the weather, or the usual topics of a nervous stranger calling another disinterested stranger. This call was all about himself which was the story of his life, so he had no trouble proceeding.

He told me after being married for nearly 50 years, he didn't love his wife. He said he never did love her. That was his opening comment. Hello!! . . . "We all knew that!!" I thought. It was rather obvious in my 17 years of association with him under the same roof with his spouse. So . . . I'm waiting for the punch line. A person doesn't get a call out of the blue from totally estranged parent for that many years unless there's some kind of a story or a mea culpa or something relevant to the DNA bond between father and son. "Maybe he's dying of cancer," I thought.

You can't make this stuff up because this is the stuff of real life. It's part of whom I am and part of this special emotional cleansing that's so significant because his soul has long departed somewhere, while my earth-bound baggage was still firmly stuck in a well-hidden do-loop of childhood confusion and subconscious silent anger dwelling on this past non-relationship between father and son until a just few days ago . . . after beginning the Teasel.

Storl talks about the Teasel being more than a bacterial spirochete killer. I'm not sure if my emotional cleanse started during the bull bellowing moment out on the grassy field or earlier in the month, just a few days after beginning the Teasel when I experienced those lightning like invisible flash sensations out of my left leg. Who knows for sure, but I definitely have been cleansed big time from some pretty significant baggage.

Storl is convinced Teasel is possibly some type of spiritual elixir that has the potential to metaphorically exorcize and cleanse stuff beyond Lyme bacteria from our depths.

Dear Reader, I'm not seeking sympathy. This is life, and any of the lifetime of unsavory thoughts or deeds or transgressions swirled into the immortal mix of life to cause this great father-son divide, and then to have experienced a singular emotional cleansing from that toxic domestic past, is the stuff of divine providence. But the 64-dollar question must be asked: "Did the Teasel help bring on this cleansing?" I think it did, because what other timely explanation can a person come up with? Scientists would call this a controlled experiment with the Teasel being the outside variable in the mix to observe in the process. I'll go with Storl and the theory that more transformative processes can occur with Teasel than just knocking down all those nasty Lyme spirochetes.

Back To The Telephone Call

So after he said he doesn't love his wife of fifty years and never did, I asked him what his next move was. He told me point blank without an emotional flinch, "I found someone who's good at cribbage." This is a 75-year-old man reinvesting his emotional quota with a cribbage lady and I thought, "This is the first time in this guy's entire life that he called me and his whole universe is rocked by a 75-year-old cribbage player so thoroughly, that he hasn't a single thing in his mind to talk to his youngest son about but his new love who is a great cribbage player."

"Holy Corona this is really getting interesting," I thought. He continued on to let me know the U-Haul was ready and he was leaving tomorrow to drive clear across the country for a brand-new life with his cribbage sweetie. I thought, "WOW, this is getting really fascinating!" Here was a long lost parent who had never spoken to his son for some 21 years on the phone, and he opens the conversation without asking him how that son is doing, or his wife is doing and begins jabbering about cribbage like nothing else matters in his life!

I was fascinated so I had to contribute at least one humanistic question aside from the cribbage story: I asked him very directly, "Have you considered your spouse? Have you considered she may jump off a bridge?" My wife is my witness; those were my exact words to him on the one and only phone call he made in his entire life to me. *"Have you considered your spouse? Have you considered she may jump off a bridge?"*

He was calling me for whatever deep psychological reasons he probably knew not himself, to tell me he had loaded up the U-Haul, and was leaving his wife for good to go shack up with his cribbage lady clean across America. That behavior actually, in this day and age, isn't something so unusual. It seems like people are always jumping ship at any age, for any reason, and some reasons are a lot more lame than finding a new card partner.

It was his interesting response to my question that took the cake and makes his call so memorable to this very day.

Here was his response to my concerns for an early September bridge jump by his spouse, my mother ... in very clear sober measured words: *"She's a tough old bird ... she can take it."* His tone wasn't haunting or vindictive, just stone cold and inhumane.

"Wow!!!" I thought. This was such a soulless inhumane response he must not have cared about anybody on the planet but himself. Here was a tax paying model, retired citizen, not some drugged out homeless drunk living under the bridge, and yet he could care less if another human being goes and kills herself by jumping off a bridge because she's a tough old bird and can take it, while he drives his U-Haul trailer off into the sunset.

Extraordinary, I thought. *"She's a tough old bird . . . she can take it?"* This was extraordinary to me, not because of his sentiments about spousal bridge jumping by the old bird, but because he called me up to express them! Most people keep pretty much quiet about that level of vitriol in their life. He must have been on the brink himself. I was a little embarrassed he chose me, a total stranger, to ooze his special departing invective puss about his wife, who was my maternal mother. Rest her poor tortured Jewish soul in peace. She must have lived in total and complete hell her entire life with such a callous piece of work. God rest her soul. May she have a good proper place in heaven.

I wished him a good life with the cribbage lady and that was the last I ever heard from him after he hung up. He died 15 years after that call and who knows where he's buried. I've not had a concern or an interest in whatever happened to that man or where he got buried . . . until just a few days ago . . . when I got a bolt out of the Teasel blue.

A few days ago during my daily morning Teasel ritual, I received one of those transmissions like I remember from the Laguna ridge-top. The very clear message was this: I need to place some dried Teasel plants on my Mother's grave, and one on my father's as well. The instant warm feeling that rolled over me was like some powerful cleansing sensation. At that moment of divine intercession, a lifelong, deeply held, and toxic foment in me was magically swept out of my system like nothing I can possibly describe. (Recall the Teasel ritual invocation . . . *cleanse my body, mind and spirit of all impurities*) . . . I could feel at that moment my battle with the paternal demons was over and done. The irrelevant son was no longer irrelevant.

Those demons simply dissolved and were done and gone for the first time in my life. Poof! Gone! "How do I feel about all that," you may ask. I feel at peace today. That's it . . . fully at peace for the first time in my life about an infected issue of domestic conflict. What a wonderful whole feeling to have a settled peaceful heart.

Last I was told after that phone call, he packed up, got a new address and phone number on the East Coast . . . so I guess he enjoyed his new cribbage life. Notwithstanding the fact that he included me on his notification list about his grand exit to greener pastures, I don't find this narrative passage gossipy or revealing of any secret family scandals considering he plowed a pretty spectacular public wake out of town upon his departure from that lifelong marriage. To me this narrative passage is my rehash of well-known public knowledge and is simply uncensored real family life, from my perspective. He's just a part of this healing story, nothing more, nothing vindictive.

Once my father was long dead, I know my mother survived it all, because I finally called her near the end of her life. My call was just another one of those bolts out of the blue. I did, and could tell she was failing. She didn't remember that her son had worked at *paradise lost* for five glorious years, from age 12 to 17. Nobody probably ever fully realized why I worked like a demon, saved every nickel of hard earned money and plotted out an escape route since I was 8 years old. She surely understood deep within her soul the pain I carried, but she likely had more than a plateful of her own overwhelming pain to manage just to survive. She said she was sorry how it all turned out. I told her not to be sorry for me and that I had lived a great and full life since I had left home. I was the lucky one, or so I thought. I was able to get out and be free, well almost free but not emotionally free until just a few days ago. I feel terribly sad for her, that a very fine descent human being had to put up with so much abuse for a lifetime. Her life must have been a living hell on earth.

I'm very thankful Mr. Teasel and whomever you're connected to in the universe for such an important emotional cleansing. I don't know how all this spiritual stuff works, other than you're a beautiful wild plant growing in a ditch beside our house hiding in plain sight. Teasel, you're my hero because I know if I hadn't found you, I'd be the one still stuck in the ditch of childhood internal foment.

She never spoke of her departed husband or whatever became of him. Her most important point she stressed to me was that her Jewish Canadian family had descended from a long Jewish lineage extending back through old France and Eastern Europe, which makes me a maternal birthright Jew. That was pretty cool news that I wish I had known years earlier. That's why I had my DNA tested to confirm my heritage, and now know that I'm an Ashkenazi Jew of deep lineage that goes back 25,000 years into the heart of the Middle East.

Maybe that was the best gift she could give and her spiritual way to expose a piece of my life's puzzle, and to help me understand all the spousal pain she held inside. Maybe that's why I needed my own Karmic trip through three years of early grade school inquisition. Maybe that was her departing soul telling me that her life was the end point to some giant round trip back through an ancient cycle where her family had been abused over hundreds of years. Who knows. I'm at peace and thankful because I feel a long era of deep pain is finally closed.

Dear Reader, as much as I purport to have some bulletproof emotional exterior, any human being is in total and complete denial if they don't think that stuff like this could eat them alive. I hope others try the Teasel for the potential emotional cleansing effect alone. I believe something special is going on with the Teasel, just like Storl suggests.

Below is a review about a book that was once very important for me. I read it more than twenty years ago. Actually, I tied to read it, but I stalled out after a couple of the case studies. I stalled out like the word "yellow" used to hit me in the solar plexus. That "yellow" stall-out feeling is beyond fear. It's pure intimidating terror to the depths of my soul and I know not why. To this day, I don't know the significance of the word "yellow", and why it used to grip me like some blacksmith's monster hot iron tongs squeezing the life force out of my body. I probably never will understand the source of the "yellow" fear.

This wonderfully insightful book was gifted to me by a kind and earnest person from Whitefish, Montana who may have herself had to deal with some personal demons. Or perhaps, she recognized my bubbling caldron, and was a messenger from the spirit forces. If ever she finds her way to this book and reads this particular passage, she'll know who she is, and I thank you for helping me on my journey. I did read the first two stories in Paul Mones' book before I stalled out in my "yellow" fear. After reading those stories, I knew where I've traveled and that I'm okay.

This is a book written by a famous defense attorney who defends children who kill their parents. The title is appropriate, *When a Child Kills*. Mones is a steadfast child advocate and trial lawyer who details in the book eight case studies of very troubled young people who murdered their parents. I believe if we study and can begin to understand the how and the why that these young children plunge over the very edge of sanity, into the absolute darkest and nastiest recesses of living hell, and when we learn how young children are able to kill their own parents, then we'll all begin to move toward a safer, less violent culture.

In a safer culture of less fear and less need to protect ourselves from the dangers that lurk in the shadows of society, away from a culture so twisted that we have created a world where young innocent children find emotional safety by killing their parents, is a less violent world I want to live, a place where young children have no "yellow" fear.

A Customer Book Review, September 15, 1997
Amazon Book Sales (Paperback Edition)
(from amazon.com)

"When A Child Kills" is an exceptionally insightful view of family violence and it's tragic outcome. Paul Mones shows us the unflinching truth of what we are doing to our children and what happens when they snap. With sensitivity for the real victims of parenticide, he describes, with numerous case examples, the various players in violent familial relationship and the almost predictable way that some children fight back.

Mones discusses how some children are abused, unloved and humiliated repeatedly until they fear and loath their own parent. This fear and loathing mixes with the love they have for the parent and they end up feeling trapped and helpless. When they can no longer take the abuse or fear so desperately the next episode, they strike out at the moment they feel safest (usually when the parent is asleep). Mones explains how the child's fear is the very thing that makes the public believe the murder was in cold blood.

I could say you won't want to put this book down but I found that I had to put it down frequently because I was shaking, I was so mad at the parents for the abuse and the untenable situation into which they put their own children.

A disturbing, well written, thoughtful, honest book.

Robert Quinn-O'Connor
robo@critpath.org
Collingdale, PA, USA

Here's The Happy Beginning

Monday, January 4, 2016, 12:00 p.m.
I've Completed This Chapter, Chapter 12

Here's a picture of that Raleigh 3-speed bike with saddlebags, all ready to roll. This is the day I assembled it out of a cardboard box. Notice the size of the front wheel and the top cross bar, in relation to my size and my step-over right leg, touching the right pedal top in bare feet. This Raleigh 3-speed definitely was an oversized bike for a bigger and older rider. I always was a big thinker planning into the future.

This photo below was taken Spring of 1963 on our front lawn when I was 11 years old... and had sold enough greeting cards door to door in the previous 18 months to earn the necessary catalogue points to ride that brand new bike into the future. That bike became my magic carpet leading to freedom. That young kid in the picture has remained steadfast and resolved up to this day, 52 years later, when that same little boy finished this Chapter 12 of his life leading right back to 1963.

At 63 years old, that little boy is still inside me today, and is thankful that he has recently become as ambitious and able to explore the world as he was back then, but is most thankful because he's now capable of living a more peaceful life he always wanted beyond the horizon of the day at hand.

I'm thankful for Dr. Halverstadt, Dr. Glidden, MR.TEASEL, and Dr. Storl. I'm thankful to you all who are part of this process, and all who are reading this story with your kind and patient understanding.

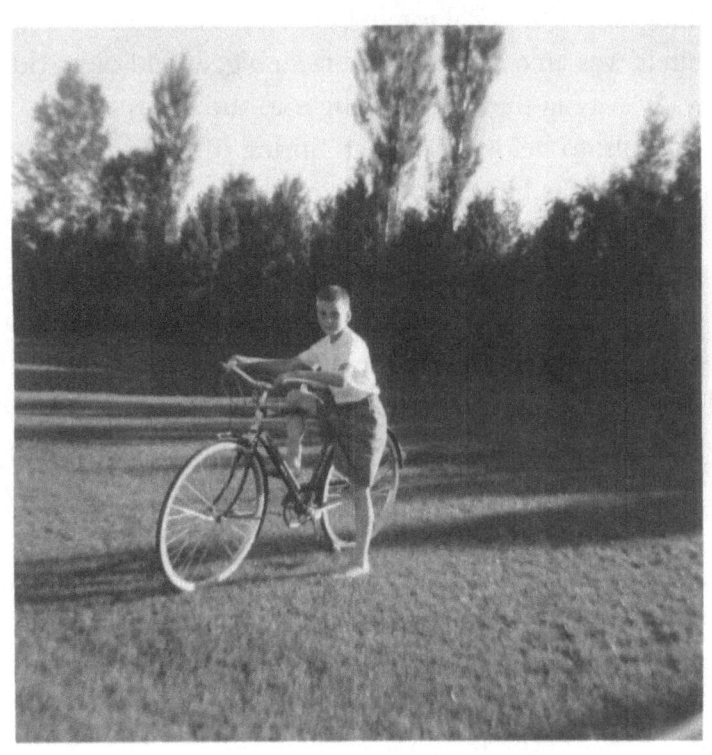

Me & My Raleigh 3-Speed Bike, Spring, 1963
© 2016 Jim Lindl

Chapter 13:
The Wild Horsetail Tea

Wednesday, January 06, 2016, 4:52 a.m.
Day 31 On The Full Cartilage & Lyme Protocol
Day 33 On The Teasel
Day 2 On The Wild Horsetail Tea
45 Days Since Beginning This Journal

I've begun drinking the Wild Horsetail (*equisetum arvense*) tea a couple of days ago to enhance the cartilage rebuilding process in my knee. This is a short, leafy type of horsetail plant that I know nothing about, except that it grows downstream on our property alongside the river under a gorgeous towering white oak.

Matthew Wood, one of the preeminent herb healing experts in the United States, states emphatically that the Wild Horsetail will absolutely help repair damaged ligament, cartilage and other connective tissues. I'm going to dive right in and read his work plus any other sources and will report in this chapter whatever looks important and useful to the process of naturopathic healing, but first, a bit of reflection on the last chapter while I sip my first daily cup of this cartilage rebuilding Horsetail.

This morning as I re-read the closing few pages to Chapter 12, it's obvious there was a significant cathartic purge in the past month. The writing tone in those passages was respectful and thankful about closure and a new beginning, about a fresh start in life. "Fine and dandy," I thought, "but what's next?"

That was yesterday and today the bills have to be paid. Today is Wednesday and this hard-nosed, ex-logger and entrepreneurial businessman is back in the reality saddle with his bum knee that's ten country miles away from being fully functional even though the Lyme spirochetes seem to be getting their butts' kicked pretty thoroughly 33 days into the fight.

The verbal, cognitive and emotional transformation in the first thirty days was profound indeed and I understand all that. I'll take it all and I'm deeply appreciative of everything that's happened. I certainly understand the merit of a sound functioning brain, and I think my lengthy chapter of review and reflection clearly indicates my brain is back and doing pretty well, possibly better than ever. I give the Teasel and the Greater Force all the credit as you know. However, my functional brain and balanced emotional state are just the foundational beginning.

I'm not Mr. Physicist who can wow the world from a wheel chair. I'm not a tournament bridge player, or a master class, chess player who can stay happily occupied in a chair at a retirement home here in France. I need mobility to get on with the life that I want to lead. I have big plans of activity and that means full mobility.

I feel right now, while sitting at the keyboard this morning, that during the immediate period leading up to December 4th, I had been the sole survivor on a slowly sinking ship without any motive power or navigational capability. Before December 4th, I felt like I was dead in the water and slowly going down and very close to the waterline. That's a fairly apt metaphor how I felt before I began this naturopathic healing journey. Dead in the water and sinking below the waves at age 63.

Over this past month since my brain woke back up and

my motivation levels and cognitive ability kicked back into high gear, I feel like the ship stopped sinking and I've got all the navigational light turned back on, but still have no motive power to continue the journey. I need motive power in my body to fully function or I'll still be dead in the water with the lights all turned on but no ability to sail away over the horizon, which is where I know I'm destined . . . somewhere over the horizon.

I feel like my mind is fully back but my body isn't keeping pace and not very useful just yet. I'm tremendously thankful I can think clearly and that a load of toxic domestic baggage vanished never to bother me again. That's all well and good, and wonderful and necessary.

However, I need my knee to giddy up under me and go. That's the resolve I have going forward: It's all about the knee cartilage from here on out. The Lyme and all its toxicity are all just about dead and buried as far as I'm concerned . . . but my body needs motive power.

Wild Horsetail will become part of that *healing equation along with the rest of the nutritional products*. Who knows if it'll do anything. We'll see, but I'm optimistic because of how well the Teasel worked out.

Skin-Sack Of Bones

There's a lot more going on with my right knee and my other joints in the past month not recorded yet, so now is the time for more details that were very present and unusual, back in mid-December but not spoken about back then. I call it the *bag of bones syndrome*. From the day I began taking the Teasel and the full protocol, both my knee joints and my hip sockets got looser and looser and looser leading up to the surgeons meeting on December 16th. During the surgeon's examination, he rotated and manipulated all my joints, both left and right sides, through a series of diagnostic motions. I could definitely feel that everything was disconcertingly loose. In fact when I walked, my hip sockets' connective tissue, or whatever holds everything together, was internally twanging and snapping around like loose sloppy rubber bands as I walked. Same with both knees. The surgeon raised his eyebrows and commented about this unusual sloppy joint condition present on both knees and both hip joints. He assured me in the surgical procedure, he could tighten up any connective tissue as required on my bum right knee.

He double checked my good left side, raised his eyebrows a noticeable second time, and asked if I had any pain with this movement, while he waggled my good knee and good left hip. He seemed surprised there was so much loose play in two good joints. There was no pain, just sloppy looseness. Very noticeable to both of us.

I had this very same sensation with both sides. It felt like all my ligaments and tendons got permanently extended far beyond their usual range of motion that I had been accustomed. It was about this same time period, mid-December, that I began easily touching down to my second knuckles when reaching for the floor. I had gained remarkably flexibility very rapidly in 11 days on this nutritional herbal protocol with no supplemental stretching. It was like overnight I was limber and nicely loose all over. In 11 days I'd become more flexible than fifteen years ago when I was climbing a high technical standard in Rock Climbing Gyms which requires significant gymnastic flexibility to mount artificial climbing walls. This new unusual flexibility didn't feel healthy or normal but it did feel transitory. I wasn't particularly concerned going into the Périgueux pre-surgery meeting.

Leading up to mid-September, for four straight months, I religiously performed all the Egoscue stretches every day for at least a full hour, usually more, and yet the flexible results that Pete suggested usually occur within a few weeks, never happened to my body. By the time of that Périgueux Surgeon's meeting December 16th, I felt like a bag of loose rattling bones in a tight skin-sack, called a human body.

My hunch, back then, is that I was rapidly dumping all the spirochetes from all the muscles, ligaments, tendons, and connective tissue and that these bacteria had been the cause of my total muscular system lock-up into a rigid mass of stiffness that caused inflexibility and diminished strength. That was my hunch, but I just wanted to wait it out before reporting these early, obviously new, and rapidly changing sloppy joint conditions in this mid-December time frame.

My intuition back then was that these loose, sloppy joints would all go away and that the ligaments would somehow re-tighten to new proper length, at some time in the future . . . that was my hope . . . and they gradually did.

That's why I'm reporting this past *Bag of Bones* condition now because it's all passed. My muscular structure cycled from complete system tightness on December 4th, to a bag-of-bones climax by late December. Today as I write, everything seems to be all snug and nicely fitting together just right. Not tight, not loose, just normal. I notice firm muscular and joint normalcy when I walk up or down the stairs, sit down in a chair, fetch some firewood, or mount the lawn tractor.

Interesting to me, is that today everything seems to be all hooked up properly, but for about two weeks in mid-

December, I thought, *if this doesn't get better, I could be in a wheel chair for the rest of my life in some late-stage syphilitic like disease state.*

I wasn't overly concerned at the time because I trusted the Teasel and trusted my body to heal properly. It all worked out okay but at the time, it was pretty weird like nothing ever experienced before in my life.

Muscular Balance Is Back

Today I can easily do all the Egoscue condition II stretches with equal balance on the right and left side. After twenty continuous weeks of intense stretching last summer, this is something I was never able to achieve I believe Lyme bacteria had a death grip on my muscular system and had it locked up tight. My system doesn't feel locked up anymore.

I also noticed that when raking up some yard leaves today, I'm surprisingly ambivalent about using a right side sweeping motion or a left side sweeping motion. Virtually ambidextrous on either side, without favoritism. That's a first in my life. I've always had a preferred work stance that utilizes motion on only one side. That preference is totally gone. Something I'll keep on the *notable list to watch.*

My intuition tells me that this chronic, muscular lock-up was probably also the cause of my diminishing physical strength over the 7-year period after I got the tick bite in 2007. My muscle tone, definition and strength are slowly coming back. It's noticeable. I notice how I can easily carry a full arm-crook of firewood into the house today, unlike five weeks ago. I expect the Wild Horsetail to encourage more proper redevelopment of all my connective tissue and that's why it's now part of the daily routine: Two cups of Wild Horsetail Tea every day. I never want to wind up like a sickly skin-sack bag of old bones. I know how haunting that syphilitic condition can feel. It wasn't good.

Storl alludes to these conditions prevalent in Old Europe during the 300-year reign of the Syphilitic Plague that began with Christopher Columbus's return from the Caribbean. His entire crew was infected with Syphilis when they returned, a disease unknown in Europe before they set sail nine months previously. That voyage to the New World changed history in more ways than I had realized before reading Storl's book on Teasel.

Friday, January 08, 2016, 11:45 a.m.
Day 33 On The Full Cartilage & Lyme Protocol

Uh Oh! Time to shift back to the Lyme symptoms. The Cartilage and Horsetail Conversation will have to wait.

So much for the Lyme bacteria being all dead and gone. The Wild Horsetail writing will have to wait until later: The lightning flashes are back.

It was 7:30 a.m. and breaking dawn this morning when I was out walking the dog, out on the 500-meter circuit, when I shook my head, testing for some lightning flashes. Those flashes all but disappeared after two days on the full protocol December 7th, thirty-two days ago.

Yep, you guessed it; all the flashes are back and very bright. About as strong and bright as before I began the protocol 35 days ago. They occur in both eyes, down in the lower outside corners in hot whitish and orange color. They're there with each firm side-to-side headshake. Shake left and both eyes fire a flash. Shake right and both eyes fire a pronounced bright flash. Every time . . . so I stopped after a good definitive test.

I'm not disappointed or concerned and let me explain why: Two days ago, the farting cycle came back, and noticeable. Not like 25 days ago when I had those staccatissimo denim ripping strings, but farts are back and noticeable. Not only are the farts back, but the stool composition changed quite dramatically as well. This elimination and farting behavior, to me, indicates additional new detoxing in progress.

This morning was the clincher. After returning from the dog walk and back into the house, a few, deep, dry, convulsive retches flew out, exactly like the lion roaring retches some weeks ago. These today came right up out of the blue this morning. Not as violent as the lion episode that rattled the valley hills, but it had the exact same voice, deep inside of me, like something needing to come out.

With this renewed dry retching and farting and with the significant change in stool composition, I know something is cooking inside of my elimination systems. I suspect not all the Lyme spirochetes have left the house of Lindl.

According to some of the literature and analysis about Lyme bacteria that I've read, it can take months to fully cook off all the nasty Lyme bacteria in a person's body. Some of the science indicates that Lyme bacteria may follow some sort of hide-and-seek 28-day lunar cycle. That's one of the reasons a person is put on a minimum of a 10 to 12-week course of super, heavy-duty antibiotic treatment, if not even longer. Not only are Lyme spirochetes tough customers to kill off, but I believe those spirochetes can corkscrew their way deep into just about every cellular crack and cranny in a person's body. Moreover, if they did all come out at once in a big overloaded flood, their toxic trash might be systemically overwhelming.

If it's true that the body's overall healing process is regulated by some God Given selective and timely processes, then this slow and repeated release of some more dead spirochete toxicity is a welcome sign that all is in order.

Friday, January 08, 2016, Later
My Current Health Status

Lightning Flashes In Full Force, Menacing Farts Recurring & Trending Stronger. Punctuated By Intermittent Gut Wrenching Dry Retches. Possibility Of Mud Slides If Current Detox Persists.

As suggested in an earlier chapter, my job is simply to observe and report the progress. This is an unexpected detour back to the lightning flashes. We'll see where it all goes in a couple more days.

Thursday, January 14, 2016
Day 39 On The Full Cartilage & Lyme Protocol

Seven days after the full body system status report above and I'm pleased to report that the coast is clear. The lightning is virtually all gone save for an occasional slight peripheral flash. A few mudslides came and went and the coughing and farting have all passed. I suspect some more Lyme bacteria have got chased out of hiding by the Teasel, and then got clobbered by immune boosting vitamin artillery. All's well that ends well . . . in my books . . . and the process of healing continues at the 6-week marker today.

Meanwhile here's another interesting piece of the healing puzzle that may help somebody if they ever journey down this naturopathic healing regime that I embarked upon 41 short days ago. A giant ganglion showed up . . . A double, golf-ball sized ganglion popped up out of nowhere. Again, I wanted to let this development play out for a few weeks to see what would happen. Would it get worse? Remain the Same? Go away? I soon found out.

Today as I write this narrative on January 14th, 2016, this monster ganglion is totally gone after showing up just a month ago.

It began to make its grand entrance right after the bull bellowing, dry retching episode on December 14th. It grew very rapidly and very large for about two weeks before it just as quickly subsided to almost nothing, only one month after it first appeared back in December. This thing grew to about the size of two golf balls squashed into an oblong, tear shaped hard object almost three inches long. This is significant. Let me explain.

The Mother of All Ganglions

This link is a helpful basic primer on understanding ganglions; not what causes them, because nobody seems to know, but what they look like and what people can do about this peculiar cyst-like condition. Ganglion Cyst (eHealthStar)

Before this personal episode with a ganglion, the only experience I ever had involved helping another person get rid of a small one on their wrist. They just laid their arm across the kitchen table while I twisted their writ and pressed down on the ganglion with my thumb. That took care of it instantly . . . but it wasn't nearly so big like what I had over the past month.

This one was located low down in the groin area right next to some important family equipment. It grew to about three inches long and was buried half inside and half outside. It definitely was noticeable. Little did I know these things could pop up in a variety of places, like the low groin area, until I read the link above. This informative article has a nicely illustrated body diagram of exactly when my whopper showed up out of the blue, beginning December 14th. The day after the Bull Bellowing and Lion Roaring episode out in the field, this groin bump started growing quickly. My initial hunch was that I had blown out the old hernia repair from three years ago. It was in almost exactly the same spot as the hernia incision, just a little bit lower, but interesting to me, as this bump grew daily, it didn't hurt of flutter like a hernia. It just got bigger and bigger and firmer and firmer each passing day. It was just plain weird, but not weird enough that I was ready for a trip back up to my local doctor for his opinion. I wasn't ready to hear I needed another hernia surgery on top of the old one.

At about the 2-week marker with this rapidly growing lump I'd finally had enough and by now was totally convinced it was my colon popping out through a new hernia rip or something else petty serious, so up to the local doctor I went. He was quite puzzled and hadn't any explanation other than reassuring me this big growing groin lump most definitely wasn't another hernia. His recommendation was an ultrasound test. It's now been ten full days since that ultra sound and the whole thing has disappeared. Poof! . . . Gone!

Round trip from nothing, to a double stacked, golf ball sized oblong ganglion, and back to zero, in one month. Something was going on down there in that groin area.

Dear Reader, these ultra sound films are a bit too personal to flash in this journal, so you'll just have to settle for my word. They were done by the same Radiologist in the same clinic as my knee x-rays back in October.

I'd love to talk with a Naturopathic Doctor about this lump growing episode. Maybe one day they can contribute to this journal with some comments.

That would be terrific because I certainly haven't a clue as to why this ganglion occurred ... but I do have a strong hunch and here is my speculation. If you backtrack to the My *Green Mile* Chapter, you'll find this passage sited below about violent convulsing and my spasmodic efforts to expel something foreign to my body ... something hidden, deep inside. This passage was written 11 days after beginning the full healing regime. Here is that 90-second spasmodic episode in its entirety.

The Bellowing Bull Returns

I was bellowing a deep dry cough like nothing ever experienced before in my life. Not sloppy phlegm, not like food crumbs going down the wrong way, not a tickle at the top ... this was deep and very dry and powerful. Like I had to expel something. Something wanted to come out but it wouldn't budge. Not up and out ... it just wanted out through my chest. Like it had to burst out of the sternum and the solar plexus region. Not up through the throat but out of the chest through the fleecy shirt and the outer jacket I was wearing ... like a Fukushima Reactor burst. I was expecting some sort of explosive force, but it never came.

I felt like that prisoner in "The Green Mile" wanting to expel something not meant to be in a human being. Something foreign needed to be pushed out. That was the coughing ... Then the nauseating dry retching began. No fluid came up, just dry retching ... even more decibels than the coughing. At first bent over and then erect, then bent over, and then erect again, and then bent over again. I bellowed like a bull moose in the woods ... very loud and reverberating off the closed in valley hills that surround our field. I'm not sure I could yell that loud. It was like I was a wounded lion roaring at the whole world around me. No anger, no fear. No emotions at all.

Then the second wave of coughing began like the first until it all stopped as quickly as it started. It was so sublimely violent it felt spiritual. None of this was painful. I actually smiled at the ridiculously unhealthy profile I must have presented in the moment. I was too convulsed to begin worrying about any of the reasons underpinning this spontaneous episode. The dog was more stunned than me and kept his distance until it all stopped . . .

My hunch is that because that groin bulge began its growth cycle immediately after that session, I believe my body was going through some sort of lymphatic pumping action to get toxic sludge moving toward some unseen exit door via certain plumbing ducts that ultimately led down into the groin area. Furthermore, I suspect the toxic debris was of such volume, that it couldn't all exit in one orderly big dump. I believe it needed some time to work itself out of my system . . . possibly to ensure that a severe detox overload reaction wouldn't occur with one violent reaction to the toxins. This is just my pure speculation.

Why do I speculate like this? Because in that entire ganglion article linked to this passage there's not one iota of reasoning where these ganglions come from or where they go to when they disappear . . . but I do know for sure, the body seems to know what to do, and how to do it, if we just let these God given natural processes play out. That's my theory about this *ganglionic cycle* over the past thirty days. But there's still more to this puzzle.

Frankincense Oil

Lately this household has become like a natural pharmacopoeia. Every few days some new herbal tincture or tea or oil or herbal book arrives. We now have dozens of exotic traditional healing items in our cupboard dedicated to natural healing. It's a fragrant sight to behold! This is who we are. We're doers in life and herbalism is the new thing in this household. While I write, my wife reads and studies plants. She's ordered every single book written by Wood, and some others. In that reading, has come understanding. These days we talk about herbs and tinctures and what they're all supposed to do for people and their maladies.

Incredibly, on our farm, we now know there to be no less than a *hundred healing herbs, plants, flowers and trees within 600 feet of this computer keyboard.* Over 100! Fascinating that all this was hiding in plain sight to someone who calls himself a journeyman organic gardener. I didn't know what I didn't know! Or course the Teasel was out in the ditch and the Wild horsetail was down steam right bedside my favorite hammock tree but those two are just the beginning. By the end of this book, I'll enumerate every single living healing thing growing on this 8-acre patch of old France.

So with that back-story it probably doesn't surprise a reader to hear that this tough knurly ex-logger is now dabbling in other healing tinctures. I had my chance to experiment with the Ganglion. I knew about the three gifts of the Magi story: Gold, Frankincense and Myrrh, but didn't have a clue what Frankincense was until two weeks ago. Yep, you guess it right. I dabbed on the Frankincense and it smells wonderfully intoxicating. It smelled like an Arabian Genie should have risen out of its little bottle containing this potent ancient healing oil. Holy Corona, once again was I learning what I didn't know. I've been completely biased against all these *girly* fragrant potions all my life. Tough-logger, macho-mountain man was my persona, not some person who dabs on Holy Oil.

So things have changed in the past month. After the Teasel kicked in over the past month, I was game to try everything. I dabbed on the Frankincense paste right after the doctor's appointment and that ganglion started going back down by the next morning. By the time I had the ultra sound done five days later, it was half the original size. Half its original size in five days! The only difference was the 3-time daily application of some ancient Jesus oil.

From that point forward, I've become a staunch believer in all things herbal. Two for two. First the Teasel, and now the Frankincense.

So this passage leaves me with a good departure point to read more about the Wild Horsetail plant, which I now have every expectation to be as effective as the first two magical wonder herbs, Teasel and Frankincense.

A Change Of Heart

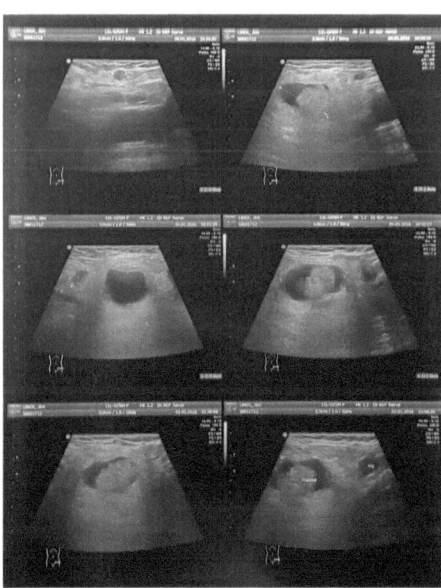

My Ganglion Ultrasound
January 05, 2016
© 2016 Jim Lindl

Like they say in Poker, "I'm all in." Well, I've had a change of heart on the Ganglion Ultrasound film. It's offered here to continue the integrity and validity of all that is written in these pages thus far. This image is "all in."

Time For More Communication With The Main Power Plant

Friday, January 15, 2016, 11:47 a.m.
Day 40 On The Full Cartilage & Lyme Protocol
Day 46 On The Teasel
Day 11 On The Wild Horsetail Tea

I've arrived at a point of realization on this 246th page of writing . . . six full weeks into this naturopathic journey. My realization is this: It's going to take some time to fully heal. I need patience. I need resolve. I need understanding that I may not get perfect knee function back again . . . ever.

I've done my part and will continue doing my part every day, but the biggest realization is this: I don't control the outcome. Greater forces out in the whirl of this vast universe are what guide and direct all human healing, and will make the difference going forward.

What I *can* control, is my desire for mediation and focus on those greater powers. I can try to commune with them in harmony. In that sublime process . . . I do believe I'll have the possibility to be fully healed but this'll take some time.

The physical, the mental and the spiritual stability of the quiet life on this farm, in this quiet period of winter, allows me to go deep into meditation for communion with these greater mysterious powers. This great whirl of cosmic energy, I'm sure, is directly connected to every single cell in my body. I need to ensure that this body of mine is fully plugged into that source of power to properly heal.

I know how this process of meditation is supposed to work. I've studied and practiced it a bit over the years. That's where I'm going for a few weeks. I'm going into the deepest of communion, to try and connect with the main Power Plant.

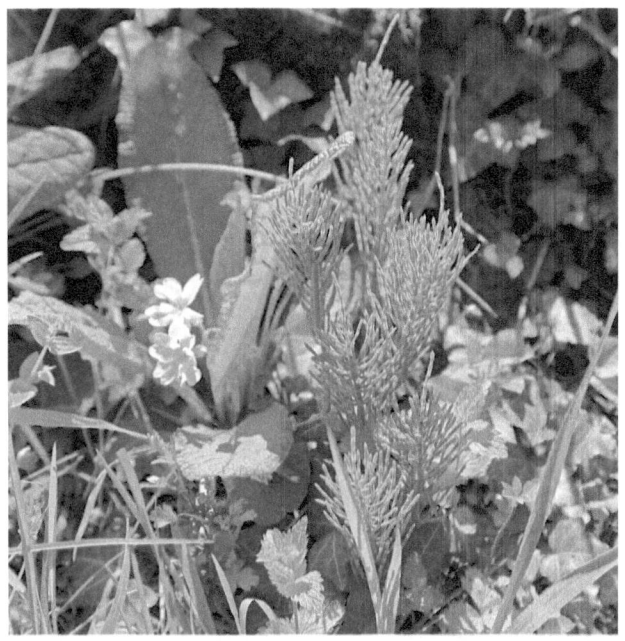

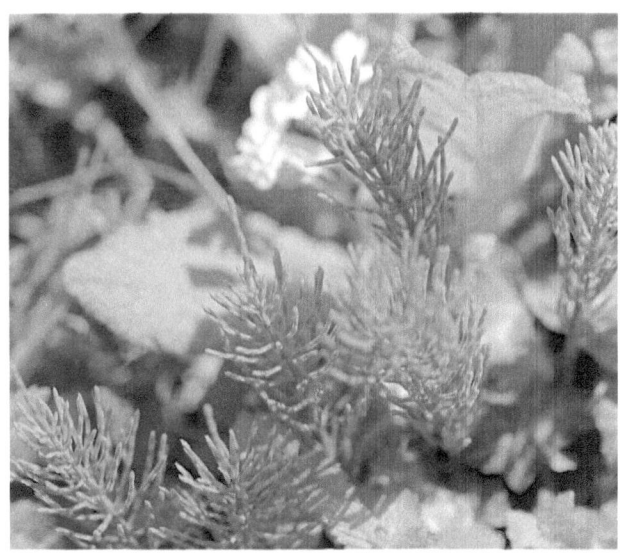

Wild Horsetail, Growing Along Our River

Chapter 14:
Voices From The Wilderness

Sunday, January 17, 2016, 10:23 a.m.

One particular voice I heard this morning didn't originate from some burning bush on a mountain near this farm while meditating. No, today's crystal clear voice came from the mountains near Denver. It came from a Doctor's keyboard in his Boulder stem cell clinic and landed in my inbox of e-mails stacked up over the weekend. Let me explain.

We all know about the *Voice* of Modern medicine on American TV. When my wife and I arrived in California this past September for my medical appointments, the very first thing I noticed different in American TV programming was the constant barrage of big pharma ads. In Europe, there are none. None, as in *Zero None*. They're banned here in Europe. In fact, big pharma ads are banned in every country in the world except New Zealand. We've watched a fair amount of French television programming to learn the language and in the eight years watching TV here we haven't seen one single drug ad, but yet, in our little village of less than 4,000 people, we have three top of the line, very nice full-service little pharmacies. It's not like we shy away from modern pharmacology and drugs. Drugs are very front-and-center in French Health Care philosophy, but only when absolutely necessary. Drugs are considered a sometime necessity, but not considered a long-term solution through dependency.

In France, TV ads are usually all about food, chocolate, perfume, and beauty, or in a different season, automobiles, travel, and sports come into vogue. That pretty well sums up our French consumptive priorities, depending on the TV season.

In America, to me, the big pharma ads felt heavy and stifling . . . they felt like unwanted brain washing with all the implied need for drugs. It actually felt *unhealthy* hearing the constant drum beat every twelve minutes about ubiquitous disease states on TV ads . . . Drugs, Drugs and more Drugs for everything imaginable. I felt saturated with drug ads after a week in America . . . and we watched very little TV in California except to catch the local news about the catastrophic 500 year drought cycle and fires.

So yes of course, there's a Modern Medicine *Voice* promoting their interest and their point of view in all variety and manner in America. I just read today, from government-compiled statistics, that all things related to medicine and medical care in America amounted to roughly 18% of the United States Gross National Product in 2014. By 2017, this large slice of the American pie will approach 20 percent with no ceiling in sight. The ceiling limitation seems to be only money, which is running a bit tight these days.

On the other hand, all the food related products, services, and food regulated crops and animals under the USDA purview, in the United States, clocks in at less than 5 percent of the Gross Domestic Product in 2014. That enormous food list includes everything from artichokes and anchovies to zucchini and Zambucca liquor. It includes all restaurants, beer gardens and pizza parlors, fast food, slow food, fish, leather, feathers, eggs, cotton, oils, grains, beer and booze, and anything we put into our mouth to eat including tobacco and candy. Even with that humongous big number, Americans spend four times *more* on health care than all that foodstuff put together. It seems like this food/medical calculus implies it's cheap to eat and expensive to get sick: Interesting equation, interesting system. Big Medicine certainly has a vocal presence in all our lives and not just in America, but they're certainly not a voice from the wilderness.

The voice that dropped into my computer mail box on the weekend was a blog post by a Medical Doctor of some note who is, by his own admission, fessing up on behalf of his entire profession, that the holistic crowd, the naturopaths the chiropractors the herbalists and the bushy-bearded ones, had some of this healing stuff right all along. He doesn't apologize for his profession's tardy understanding about how the human body actually works in the healing process, but he does admit that the old-fashioned holistic crowd had it right over this past century and that his establishment group is just catching on, according to a *scientific study*.

So what's this big wilderness truth you ask? It's exactly this . . . and this simple: *The body can and will heal itself, including cartilage in knee joints!* That admission of truth by a medical study is like admitting there's a Supreme Being by an atheist. This admission, this *finding* by the medical community is huge and we should embrace them, not ridicule them.

There's a lot of room at the back row holistic pew in the holy cathedral of modern medicine. It's been a hundred lonely years for the naturopaths, the chiropractors, and the herbalists. Very lonely indeed. These natural healers have barely squeaked out a tiny voice in this church while someone else ran the pulpit sermon up front.

This self-healing business is holy doctrine writ large of naturopathic philosophy and this *Voice From The Wilderness* that landed in my inbox is singing loud and clear that it's time for a shift of thinking by his establishment medical colleagues.

This Doctor's daily blog and the attendant scientific study embedded in the link below indicates this trend of thinking may be finally appearing on the horizon. Hallelujah for the health of everybody if we embrace this truth. This Doctor is pretty excited about this direction of scientific discourse. This is what his stem cell clinic is all about: Self-healing with some technical assistance. This type of discourse opens up the possibility that a whole new army of Medical Doctors may come over to our camp for good reason: Stem cell healing works on knees, which to me, is a logical bridge to then ask . . . what other areas of the body can heal because of its wonderful God-given self-healing design? I think maybe just about everything! That's what my Teasel experience is telling me.

That's exactly what my knee cartilage re-growth program is all about: Self-Healing. I've just decided to skip the bone drilling and the extractive procedure into my hip to draw out a pea-sized dab of my own cells to kick things off. According learned sources, my knee cartilage re-growth success will have a good chance on its own as long as I give it a boost with the daily nutritional artillery barrage. We'll see how this route all works out. I'm almost seven weeks into the program and I can walk with a lot less pain. That's my holistic experiment in its essence: Self - generating knee cartilage via my own remaining stem cells on a terribly worn out knee joint. It seems to be working out so far.

This is what my Lyme disease eradication program is also all about: Self-healing . . . with some natural assistance by the Teasel and a nutritional boost of the immune system . . . Non-surgical, non-pharmacological intervention. Natural assistance: Things like better food, some high-powered vitamins and minerals, some healing herbal tonics, good clean air and water, some yoga and some yogurt.

It's my hope that maybe we're on the cusp of new thinking and ready to shed some old biases. Maybe the time is now and we're becoming a *collective* gathering storm of realization that the recent Allopathic, Pharmacological paradigm over the past hundred years is not entirely the optimal path to vibrant health. Maybe just maybe, we'll hear even more voices from the *Establishment Wilderness* in the future. Knee Arthritis, Heal Thyself? New Research Says Yes! (Regenexx)

Knee Arthritis, Heal Thyself? New Research Says Yes!

Quote from this blog site: "Science continues to support the more than century old ideas of chiropractors and naturopaths that the body can repair itself if the practitioner creates the proper environment to facilitate healing."

Below is the second voice from the Wilderness, collectively asking the lawmakers in America to diminish big pharma's presence on public advertising by none other than the *American Medical Association* at a doctors' convention in Atlanta, Georgia, in November, 2015.

Maybe these Medical Establishment voices of reason have had enough and are ready to walk-back their medical philosophy a few decades when we actually had slimmer waistlines, simpler unadulterated foods and more affordable health care than we have today. This article below seems to indicate exactly that trend of thinking . . . maybe just maybe.

Call For Ban On Direct Consumer Prescription Drug Advertising, AMA, November 17, 2015

Interesting to me how I found this article on the 17th of January and the article itself was publicly released on the 17th of November. That number 17 shows up often for me at the most, *intersecting*, turning points in time. Number 17 means nothing to me in particular, however I do speculate that it may be something for me to note, but what? I don't have a clue. I just try to keep my eyes peeled for more directions and turning points on the journey.

Many Voices From The Wilderness

Finally, for the first time since beginning this lengthy journal almost two months ago, I'm absolutely certain a brain wave, directly from the Main Power Plant, hit me this morning. Here it is . . . in its entirety:

**This Journal Story Needs Embedded Reader Comment To Become An Accurate And Fully Relevant Read.
This Was My Bolt Out Of The Blue While Meditating.**

At this juncture, if somebody has actually invested the many hours necessary to plow through all these pages, they surely have some thoughts about something written so far. Maybe it's a Chiropractor, a Medical Doctor or a natural healer of some genre who's been itching to jump in and say, "Wait just a minute, have you thought about this?" Maybe it's somebody with Lyme symptoms. Maybe a Teasel acolyte like I've become. Maybe it's just somebody that landed on this lengthy story by accident and feels, "This is all wild and crazy," but wants to comment.

It's my hope that if somebody feels the urge to speak out they'll feel compelled to rattle the keyboard in response. I believe that by reading this far, every reader should feel that they've earned the right to take the stage and be heard by others. They can come out of the wilderness and be a voice for others to ponder on these pages. Everybody has something important to contribute. I want this Chapter 14 to become their stage to speak out. Let me explain how that can happen.

I look at this book not unlike a Bed and Breakfast Inn, with the doors wide open to the public. This book, to me, is like a friendly residence and the name of the place is called *MR.TEASEL My Hero*. You've paid the e-book tariff for a read and by paying, that tariff entitles you to spend any amount of time at this very personal residence of decorated pages. You've been politely listening to the owner's story if you've gotten this far, and like any cordial and friendly B&B, once the guests stay a night or two and chat with the other guests and owners, they've not only earned the right to comment in the guest book, but their comments are always most welcome and can be enjoyed by all who'll come and visit in the future.

The richness of any B&B grows with the participation by the patrons. I believe visiting guests usually leave a bit of their soul behind for others to experience in all the very best B&B's. My wife and I choose B&B's over other types of accommodation because they very often can have an accumulative collective personality that radiates through the owners. It's not the decoration that makes a great B&B to me, it's the vibration in the walls of the place from all those that have passed through before and infused their world into the world of the resident owners. A rich and storied B&B can introduce a guest to a world of different experiences because the owners, through their guests influence, have had contact with the outside world beyond their own *wilderness*. What comes around . . . goes around in a B&B and is enjoyed by everybody who walks through the doors if they like to chat and explore the stories of others.

That's what I hope this Chapter 14 will eventually become: A guest book of comment and discourse, a place for a nonjudgmental conversation and a meeting place of *Many Voices From the Wilderness*. That would include you, Dear Reader, if you're ever so inclined to post some thoughts . . . today, tomorrow, or maybe after you've had your own Teasel experience.

The door is open to express thoughts, questions, or ideas, corrections or amplifications . . . the possibilities are endless. The only etiquette I request is the same etiquette tradition in a guest book at a refined Bed & Breakfast: Respect, positive helpful contribution, honesty, sincerity and appropriate brevity. Maybe you want to include where you're writing from and what you do for a living, just to add some zing and zang to your post. In the weighty subjects of this Teasel Book, a person's guest book writing could run a thousand words I suppose . . . or maybe a half dozen would get the job done.

With an e-book, the addition of comments can be added on the fly or deleted, if requested, in real time. With a real time e-book communication platform, all past readers can keep abreast of *Fresh Voices* in this Chapter 14 by simply logging onto the ongoing updated versions, to read about any new fresh comment and thinking coming in from the wilderness. Everything will get posted in date sequential order, with a general subject index for an easy keyword search. If this book eventually expands to another 2,000 thousand pages . . . Hurray, hurray for being inclusive, not exclusive. It could all be searched and browsed by subject, person, title, or skipped entirely. The reader's in charge of the depth and pace of discovery to learn what's on people's minds out in the *Wilderness*.

I suspect there's the possibility that this recorded public discourse I propose for Chapter 14, could become by far the most valuable aspect of this entire book. It's quite possible this book could become a springboard for clearer and deeper understanding far beyond the limited initial links unearthed by myself as presented on these pages.

I know there's more coming in this book. My knee demands it. The Denver Doc has a scientific study that gives my holistic cartilage approach a medical blessing of approval. "Why not me, and why not now?" I ask.

"Is this all delusional thinking? Is this all just a waste of time?" I ask myself. I don't think so. One thing for sure that's not a delusion is the Teasel and my Lyme symptoms getting annihilated after thirty days on the protocol.

Teasel is a beautiful plant growing 250 yards down the road from us and it sure seems to have done amazing things for me. It was hiding in plain sight and I didn't have a clue two months ago, that a healing solution was right here under my nose. That is fact, not delusion. So I expect there's at least one kernel of truth in all this verbose writing so far. I hope to add more and with the help from other voices, maybe many more truths can be uncovered for all of us readers.

Chapter 14, A Public Place For Voices In The Wilderness To Share Their Thoughts To The Spine Of This Book's Central Story: Teasel, Lyme, Cartilage And General Self-Healing. This Was My Bolt Out Of The Blue Today.

If you'd like to post a comment in this designated public arena of kindred souls, *"Many Voices From The Wilderness"*, about virtually anything, anonymously or with a partial name, where you are writing from etc., it'll be most welcome. Contact me at ..... *this sentence was never completed in the final edited edition because...*

Editor's note:

At this juncture of Jim's writing he had not considered the possibility of setting up a dedicated website with a full featured blog for the public to write the type of input and discourse he envisioned. That website and blog capability of course has been built at mrteasel.org *as part of the Non-Profit Teasel Foundation.*

Chapter 15: Bowen Technique, Bowen Therapy

Thursday, January 21, 2016, 2:30 p.m.
Day 46 On The Full Cartilage & Lyme Protocol
Day 52 On The Teasel
Day 17 On The Wild Horsetail Tea
Day 4 On The Wild Horsetail Tincture
Day 3 On The Mullein *(verbascum thapsus)* Tincture *(new)*
61 Days Since Beginning This Journal

When I woke up this morning, the very first thing I thought about was Bowen Therapy. The Bowen Technique was a fairly obscure modality of healing not well known outside of Australia until the last decade or so, but in Australia, this body-mechanical, body-touch technique is probably as well-known as Chiropractic care and for good reason. Tom Bowen was an Australian who developed this total body healing technique and his ideas have spread worldwide because of the hundreds of thousands of people who personally swear by its magical effectiveness. Many of them became true believers because, when nothing else worked, this obscure last resort healing art came and rescued them from their misery and pain. I've personally met quite a number of these Bowen Believers when I lived in Northern California. Back in my vitamin business era, I ran into all sorts of interesting people

... established credible people ... honest sincere leaders of our community who privately led me to different areas of health and healing that I had no idea existed. Bowen Therapy was one of them and I tried it for my chronic neck and back pain that's been with me for an adult lifetime. Unfortunately, the Bowen Technique never worked for me.

I'm not personally one of these fervent Bowen Believers. I tried the modality for a good two dozen treatments and it did little, if anything, for me ... but am I skeptical? Not in the slightest. I've met too many people who had amazing results from Bowen. The practitioner I worked with just couldn't seem to connect with my particular ailments. Let me explain more about what I know about Bowen and how this all comes back to the Teasel Elixir and Horsetail Tea ... and maybe most importantly ... the *Mullein tincture* which I began taking only two days ago.

The Bowen healer I used to see up in the foothills of Northern California, according to his clients, was a Bowen guru. He was a Bowen teacher who ran acclaimed workshops as well as a dedicated practitioner five days per week. They said he was probably one the most gifted practitioners in the United States, and from the constant stream of clients always waiting in the drawing room of his house, they were probably right. I got to know him and Bowen healing firsthand. I saw his clientele come and go from his house in all shapes and sizes, and from all walks of life. A total cross section of America demographics came to his home for treatment on his massage table in a small back bedroom. Later I learned this man was one of the earliest Bowen Acolytes who brought the Bowen Technique to the United States decades ago. I can understand why others claimed he was good. It was from him, over long and interesting conversations across his kitchen table, that he educated me about the inner workings of Bowen and what Tom Bowen had discovered by accident in Australia many decades ago. Here's what this guru told me about the mysteries of muscle memory and trauma.

Traumatic Memory Can Be Locked Deep Into Our Muscles

What this foothill's Bowen teacher claimed, is that when the human body experiences some sort of trauma, either psychological trauma or physical trauma, or a combination of both, that experience is indelibly imprinted into our muscular structure. This deep-seated resident past memory or physical traumatic imprint can lay deep and dormant for years, lurking to cause trouble at any time . . . or it can stay ever close to the surface and play havoc with our daily health. These ever-present *memories* of old are hidden deep in cellular structure never to go away . . . at least that's my understanding from our conversations. He told me that these traumatic memories will stay put, until they're dealt with in some fashion. That's only a small part of the Bowen Theory of chronic malaise. Tom Bowen, the gifted Australian self-taught healer found out about these deep tissue issues, and how to root them out through a very unique massage-like manipulation. These trouble making muscle memories can cause terrible chronic health repercussions, according to this guru educating me, while he chain-smoked oily unfiltered cigarettes at his kitchen table, twenty years ago.

He was a character for sure, but he had endless clientele who were credible human testimony that something significant was happening on his back room massage table. I was witness to it all and found him to be a fascinating personality, if not a bit quirky. Genius doesn't seem to need public decorum to cut a credible path through conventional biases. He certainly didn't. He was one of a kind and danced to a different drummer. He has since then passed away. Fair Oaks Bowen Therapy

"So why do I bring all this back-story into this book?" you're probably asking at this juncture. Well here's the point: For the past four decades since I've had my back surgery, there's one super-conscious body movement I've never been able to shake off . . . turning over in a bed while sleeping. When I sleep, like most people, from time to time I like to switch sides or simply reposition. How many times do you suppose an average person does that in forty years? Five times per night? Ten times per night? One to five thousand times per year? In 40 years that could clock-in at upwards of 200,000 body-bed turns since my surgery, back in December, 1976. That's a lot of bed shifting that I'd bet not a single person would ever give a second conscious thought about . . . unless you had a nagging fear of getting an excruciating painful back spasm by turning in bed. That would be me. That's a part of my chronic back condition . . . a nagging fear of crippling back spasms, particularly when I'm relaxed in bed.

Fear about each and every one of those individual bed-turns for 40 continuous years, was me. Every single turn . . . bar none. Every single turn or rise out of bed I've had to lock up my central torso by squeezing my butt cheeks and crunching my abs in unison and then would make the maneuver to change position or to get out of bed. It was *fear, and fear alone* that caused me to always do this muscular pre-roll procedure. It didn't matter if I had to get out of bed at three in the morning to pee. Before I'd roll out and sit up, I had to lock up the core muscles both front side and back side . . . ever since Christmas, 1976. If I didn't do that procedure, there was the potential to lock-up with a debilitating back spasm of incredible pain. I had that fear every day of my life until this morning.

Whenever I'd visit a chiropractor for treatment, uncountable times over the past forty years, I'd often comment about the fear I had of my lower back going into spasm. It was just something I lived with, even though only a very few times did my back ever lock up with a full spasm after my surgery. Maybe ten times in forty years . . . ten times at most, but the pain is so excruciating it's never forgotten. It returned just often enough, once every few years, that it was always feared like no other pain. Almost as feared as the word "yellow" described in Chapter 12.

One of these spasms hit my back last April, out in our orchard, while on my knees digging out a dandelion. Yes, Dear Reader, digging out a poor little dandelion! It hit me with full force like the Edmonton days. I collapsed and couldn't move. Three days later, it finally subsided, but in those three miserable days, I was virtually bedridden all day and all night. The slightest wrong twitch would send torture chamber daggers into my lower back. Toilet duty . . . I'll not describe. It was disgusting. I purposely didn't eat so I wouldn't have to poop. I just peed into empty one and a half liter plastic water bottles, while I lay in bed.

That was the first spasm in probably the last 15 years, and it was awful. Total spastic lock-up. Incredible pain with the slightest movement. Fearful actually. I was convinced I'd soon be in Bordeaux for a spinal back fusion. I wasn't quite ready to call the ambulance just yet, but pretty close. After three full days it released and most interestingly, it was one simple bridging static Egoscue supine stretching position for about 20 minutes, that got it all unlocked just about the time I was ready to call the ambulance. That was one scary, 3-day episode. That's when I cracked open Pete's book given to me ten years earlier by Doctor Blanchard in California. I was desperate for something. That final back spasm in April is what got me motivated to begin seriously trying to once again figure out the root of my 40-year chronic back troubles. Little did I realize in April that I also had Lyme disease attacking me at the same time. What a mess.

Yes, Doctor Blanchard is the gifted one. *The guitar picking, golf pro, chiropractor* is Doctor Blanchard. Usually all his patients call him Doctor B. I'm not disrespectful, quite the contrary . . . it's just my quirky way with doctors. In private, I usually call all DCs, NDs, MDs, PhDs, and Dentists by their first names. I always have . . . ever since a family dentist reprimanded me in front of a bunch of us 12 year olds at his daughter's birthday party to never call him MISTER so and so.

I very respectfully said hello Mister so and so . . . as we entered his mansion for his sixth grade daughter's birthday party. He said, "You will call me DOCTOR when you talk to me." Wow! I was set for life about Doctors from that birthday party onward. I never called a Doctor, DOCTOR, after that night unless it just accidentally slips out. I willfully refused to be intimidated by Doctors from that day forward. My quirky attitude was further triple whammy reinforced by one other MD in that same era of *god Doctor* mentality to forever seal my bias about American MD personality disorder. They may have thought they were gods back then, even if they didn't believe in a Deity. Pretty interesting philosophical confusion There isn't *One*, but yet they are *One* . . . I jest of course. I fully realize introductory Deity 101 was an optional class for all first year med students back then, but I was told . . . it was a highly popular elective.

I know it's all changed today, but that era of high-handed medical arrogance still sits in my craw. The Teasel hasn't cured that bias . . . yet. I still don't give any MDs a pass until they prove themselves as compassionate human beings. The linked Payola article a few chapters back, continues to fuel my bias.

Chiropractors, and other healing modalities automatically have my respect, no matter who they are or what level of competence they've achieved or what they charge. They all have my respect for one simple reason . . . they respect that I'm an equal fellow human being. I have firsthand experience with the medical community wrath that was heaped on the Chiropractic profession 40 years ago in Canada. When I got out of my back surgery, the follow-up physician, not the surgeon Dr. Allen whom I have great respect for, but the follow-up physician, made a point of telling me to steer clear of Chiropractors. "They're all dangerous quacks," he said when I inquired if he knew of one that I could see post-surgery. Social injustice is a big deal with me. It's possible the Teasel is amplifying that philosophical tendency within me. Who knows. I just don't tolerate social injustice well. Never have.

With this herbal healing I'm experiencing, there might be some attitude cleansing, but it's also possible there might be some attitude-strengthening going on as well: Physically, mentally, emotionally, and spiritually. I can feel a little bit of them all getting stronger and more defined as I write and think about these past few weeks.

The following memoriam is about a storied Albertan who

drove heavy equipment at a coalmine in his summers working his way through medical college. He and I related pretty well before and after he cut open my spinal column: British Columbia Timber Faller meets Alberta Coal Man at the operating room. In Memoriam, Dr. Peter R.R. Allen, An Albertan Neurosurgeon (1932-2013) by J Max Findlay (The Canadian Journal Of Neurological Sciences, November 2013)

From this day forward, I'll make sure I always address Doctor B. publicly as Doctor Blanchard because I'd never want anybody to interpret my casual breezy style to be anything less than the utmost respect for him. He's just completed a first draft pre-read of the first fourteen chapters of this manuscript. I trust him with my life and my heart. I consider him a confidant in all things written on these pages before the public ever reads anything here. If this rambling journalistic account passes muster with Doctor Blanchard, I know it'll be acceptable to publish one day. I feel privileged for his comments as he reads through these chapters as they're being written. Doctor Jeff Blanchard DC is a healer extraordinaire. He's a gifted one. That's why my wife and I incurred seven thousand dollars in travel expenses and endured 31 hours of arduous international travel to see him in California for a couple of thirty minute orthogonal treatments on my atlas.

Here is a link to an informative 8-minute video that describes Atlas Orthogonal principles. There are hundreds of wonderful chiropractors across America with deep experience in this powerful Chiropractic modality. Dr. Halverstadt and Dr. Blanchard are two of the best with this highly technical healing approach. Atlas Orthogonal Introduction Video (YouTube)

Back To The Back Spasm Problems

I'm sure I've had this life long, nagging, lower back fear because of my lower back surgery, but also because those types of back spasms were common for the three months leading up to the surgery.

It was during those three pre-surgery months that I was heavily medicated on Valium to prevent going into automatic spasm. Even on that powerful muscle relaxant, it wasn't unusual for me to literally collapse onto the ground, unable to continue walking until the spasms subsided. Sometimes twenty minutes would pass before they would subside and I could get up and walk. It was awful. It was incredibly painful. That went on for three full months, during October, November and December, 1976, until I literally couldn't walk any more. That's when I finally called the hospital for Dr. Allen to operate on my back. That's when they came and got me from my apartment on the 17th floor overlooking the hospital. Six days later the spasms were no more, but for the following post-surgery and for forty years . . . the fear of those spasms never left me, especially when I slept.

Experiencing those spasms on public sidewalks in subzero icy Edmonton, Alberta, in full view of gawking university students, probably ranks as an indelible experience that could be called . . . somewhat traumatic. Even for a tough-as-nails timber cutter, those were a rough three months leading up to surgery.

My muscles probably recorded those episodes and didn't want any part of them returning. I know that my brain sure remembers them like yesterday. It's also the how and the why I joined a university fraternity. One kind student used to help me through those spastic episodes while I was prostate on the ground and locked-up on icy Edmonton sidewalks. I'll never forget those incidents. We eventually became close university friends and DKE Brothers. I'm forever thankful to him and that College Fraternity.

They were both pivotal turning points in my life. College and the Fraternity friendships are what got my life redirected out of the remote Canadian West Coast logging camps. The Dekes were a perfect fit for my rough-cut insular personality. Most of them in the Edmonton Chapter were all pretty rough-cut renegades themselves . . . in their own individual ways and I fit right in. That's what the DKE is famous for: Some outstanding individual men who have created their own unique powerful dance in their life and their career. Some are legendary stories . . . astronauts, presidents, rags to billionaire rogues, like Teddy Forstmann, the Billionaire, who endorses Peter Egoscue in his book. He's a Deke. Some Dekes are the unusual suspects of history books. There's a DKE flag planted on the moon by Deke Bean. That's exactly right: There are two flags on the moon. The USA flag and a DKE Rampant Lion flag. There's a lot of Dekes in that renegade book of life. I'm still working hard on my contribution to uphold that cherished reputation. Alan Bean's Deke Moon Flag, DKE News, August 25, 2014

That lower back fear ended this morning. This morning, for the very first time in almost forty years, I was dumfounded that I could roll to either side on the bed and never gave a second thought about tightening up my core muscles. I experimented several times for validation. Poof!! Gone!! This deep residue fear factor was just not present today. Profound indeed. I just didn't seem to need that multi-decade mental preparation and protection anymore for simple body turning in a bed. My torso felt loose and flexible. It felt *safe* for the first time in forty years since that L4-L5 surgery I had at the UofA hospital. What an incredible feeling to not fear moving in bed!

I suspect that along with my emotional cleansing discussed back at the end of Chapter 12, there must have been further, "Bowen-Like" deep tissue trauma release. I'm positive something like that has happened. What else could explain this new fear-free flexibility? The daily spiritual meditation ritual? I don't think so.

Yes, the spiritualists may suggest that possibility: *"May the divine essence of the cosmic infuse my being and cleanse my body, mind and spirit of all impurities . . ."* yada, yada, yada . . . but I've been using that very same pre-meditative invocation since September, 1996. I've carefully recorded and archived a dozen handwritten spiral notebooks over seven consecutive years of serious deep spiritual meditations, and it was always the same opening ritual . . . but my back never gave up its fear. That's a ton of invocations and contemplation, but yet this specific 4-decade back trouble remained. So I don't think it was the most recent 60 days of meditative invocations asking for more cleansing that unlocked my back, although it may have helped.

So was it the Teasel Elixir? It's possible. What else has changed in my life recently that could be the causal factor? But I've been using the Teasel for seven straight weeks and had no fear-release about my back going into a spastic pain state, so probably not the Teasel, I thought. The Horsetail? Maybe that's the herb that has the magic healing power to facilitate traumatic toxic memory cleansing embedded deep within some hidden muscle groups and connective tissues. Horsetail is supposed to be good for healing all manner of damaged tissue areas in the entire muscular and bone structure. But I've been using that for three weeks also, with no big back release.

Was it the addition of the Mullein tincture? I definitely think it's the most likely candidate for this lower back fear release. One herbalist calls Mullein . . . "The Spine Straightener." Okay . . . pretty crazy . . . I know, but he said it, not me.

Maybe this Mullein plant has the necessary, vibratory characteristic to dissolve resident psychological toxicity in our bodies that lies in our muscles like the Teasel did with my brain. Who knows about all these healing mysteries, but only fifteen dollars for a month supply of tincture . . . why not give it a try? What's there to lose? Fifteen bucks? The loss is not trying it for a month. My wife is the one doing most of the extensive supplemental reading on all these new herbal concoctions arriving weekly at our house. Interestingly, mullein also grows on our property. It has a broad leafy base and then, in later summer, it shoots up a singular tall green stalk with pretty bright yellow flowers.

I sometimes wonder how on earth did these herbalists try all this stuff for the very first time and figure out all this healing truth from a bunch of plants most of us would call weeds? Pretty incredible to me how all this obscure herbal knowledge was mainstream thinking only 150 years ago and today it's virtually lost to all western populations, except to an obscure group of bushy-bearded hobbits living on the edge of "respected" civilization. Obviously, I jest. I'm beginning to feel like Storl and Wood, and other highly learned herbalists, whom are more akin to modern day holistic medical prophets out in the wilderness with their true voice of reason . . . are speaking to us lost frightened sheep . . . locked in a modern day medical insane asylum run by a bunch of state protected money grubbers.

I'm seeking input for Chapter 14. I'm seeking voices from the wilderness, written commentary by readers who also use herbal remedies and have solid knowledge in these matters. I'd love to compare notes on this particular aspect of the Mullein to further verify my hunch about Bowen-like traumatic memory cleansing results, using herbal therapy with both Mullein and Wild Horsetail. I hope somebody who has read this passage will respond someday with their knowledge and hopefully correlated experiences. I know this isn't just blind dumb luck that I can now roll out of bed without cringing in silent fear of back spasms.

The Grand Finale With The Mullein

Monday, February 01, 2016
Day 57 On The Full Cartilage & Lyme Protocol
Day 63 On The Teasel
Day 28 On The Wild Horsetail Tea
Day 15 On The Wild Horsetail Tincture
Day 14 On The Mullein Tincture
72 Days Since Beginning This Journal

Here is the drop-dead showstopper to this whole chapter:

When I took the 2oz. Mullein drink . . . during my meditative moment of contemplation . . . when I drank the 15 drops of mullein in water . . . an electrifying, almost orgasmic shiver ran from the base of my spine right up into my skull.

Nothing painful, and very short duration, but it was an enormously huge shiver . . . like the shiver a person might experience right before a flu bug, or some other nasty bug gets hold of their system. That's how this shiver felt, but in triple full house spades.

It happened two mornings in a row during a series of seven positive breathing movements while holding the glass of water with the Mullein tincture in my hands

This is all getting pretty interesting to me . . . pretty remarkable how much has transpired in such a short period of time. I suspect it's all in the vibrations of our maladies resonating with the vibratory signature of the healing herb. At least that sounds good to me. What else can it be? Maybe a voice from the wilderness can enlighten us all.

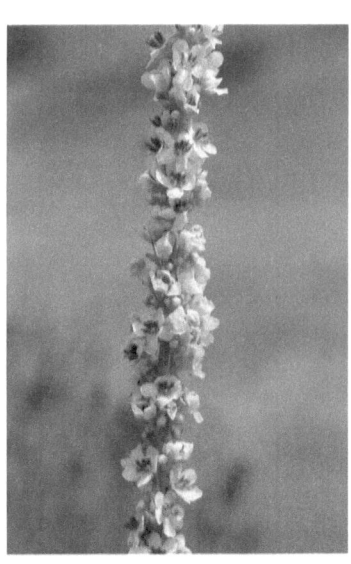

Dark Mullein Wildflowers
At Our Farm
July, 2014

Sunday, February 07, 2016
Important Postscript on Mullein

This Mullein wilderness voice just came in from the Internet!!

The Internet is such a wonderful thing. I wasn't satisfied ending this chapter last week with both the reader and myself hanging on this magic mullein business. Well, Dear Reader, click onto this link below and have a feast of Mullein pie from one of the newer bushy-bearded ones! He's an American self-taught herb healing man out of rural Michigan. This link goes to his website to enlighten us all about mullein and other things herbal. I'm beginning to feel the pull of this herbal world and I'm becoming stronger each day. It feels like the rising tide of my writing and focused study sessions within this Teasel journal is pulling my very spirit out into some great ocean of truth just waiting to be discovered.

This Michigan Herbal Man has also had a chronic bad back, and it was mullein tinctures and treatments that got him back up and running much like my own almost miraculous results. It's all in his website in great detail for the eager reader. I now realize I'm not some zany voice from the asylum of babbling herbal-healing hopeful fools.

After a person reads the "A Bit About Me" on this Michigan Herbal Man's website, I think his voracity is self-evident. Jim McDonald, Herbalist - Mullein (herbcraft.org)

What I'm beginning to feel, is a deep need to learn the truth about healing . . . and not just personal health and healing. I feel like Mr. Teasel's author has transitioned from a simple reporter on the effects of this nutritional artillery barrage and Teasel Elixir on this Jim character, to becoming an active scout seeking new routes to even bigger truths lying over the horizon. Truths I know not what, but there are more truths out there to uncover before this journal is finished.

I suspect this Mr. Teasel journey, which I began in California last September, is leading me wherever I need to go for my own healing. The Lyme disease and the bum knee were just the doorway to enter into the wilderness. I can now see that very clearly. My lower back improvement and the recent mullein experience is evidence of this suspicion. I'm sure there's more to come.

Chapter 16:
Age 64

Wednesday, February 03, 2016, 10:27 a.m.
Day 59 On The Full Cartilage & Lyme Protocol
Day 65 On The Teasel
Day 30 On The Wild Horsetail Tea
Day 17 On The Wild Horsetail Tincture
Day 15 On The Mullein Tincture
74 Days Since Beginning This Journal

It's been two weeks since my last entry in this journal. Yesterday, February 2nd, was my birthday . . . I turned 64 years old. It was good day. My older brother wrote me his annual note. In recent years, once a year, he writes a sentence or two . . . always on my birthday. That's it, but it's special. We were close when I was very young. We did a lot of exceptionally cool brother-brother things, but he moved away early . . . under different circumstances than mine. He had a big-brother influence in my early childhood. He introduced me to book learning. Lots of books. Books were his world back then. Mine was a strawberry farm. He taught me about the subatomic whirl at age 10 and introduced me to Ayn Rand and *Atlas Shrugged* by age 14.

He and I drove his car, in August, 1965 from Durango, Colorado to Chicago, Illinois via route 66, before the era of Interstate highways. I was age 13. He had just turned 19. In Amarillo, he *tried* to eat a 72-ounce steak, a huge baked potato and all the trimmings in one hour. It was free if he could wolf it down in less than 60 minutes. I had to drive after that meal. He and I thought it was nothing unusual about me behind the wheel plowing down the open road while we talked. We were open road brothers each destined somewhere back then. He did all the cities. I did some long two lane stretches down route 66 in an old Ford Falcon. My traveling money came from a glorious full summer on the strawberry farm. I was in training for something back then . . . but I knew not what . . . maybe just maybe, as I tap out these keystrokes . . . I'm beginning to figure it all out.

He taught me how to make copper pipe bombs using farmer match heads and shotgun shell powder. He made a trip to the ER because one had a short fuse that I lit too close to the base. Copper shrapnel can get nasty while tossing hand-held bombs.

He was an inquisitive scientist at an early age. He was 17 when he pulled out . . . valedictorian of his class who took the high road to high places. His destiny was set with scholarships. I didn't make it past 11th grade, and just barely managed that accomplishment. My destiny was set with a 6-10 McCulloch chain saw, and a loaded pick-up truck headed to the wilderness mountains at age 17. I've seen him maybe ten times in fifty plus years. He'll be age 70 soon.

I guided him to the Shasta Summit one spring. A good trip by all. Six of us made high camp at the top end of Giddy Giddy Gulch on that trip. I gave everybody a professional mountain snow school with big traverse exposure on the Shasta West Face below the *gendarmes*, a 1,500-foot vertical drop. That was their warm-up orientation to the summit the following day. I knew if they could handle a 42-degree high-angle ice crust with crampons and ice axes, facing a bottomless death-slide, all roped together . . . as a warm-up . . . they were ready for the hard 12-hour push to the summit the following day. That was their pre-climb test. My dentist was also on that trip. I like introducing people to nice things. Pristine alpine mountaineering or decorative Christmas cards . . . nice things. I'm a promoter at heart.

Five of us summited on that trip. One was not ready to climb above high camp. That happens. A proper and worthy guide must help each climber match their desire with their ability. He was relieved to stay in high camp and didn't feel embarrassed about his mid-mountain achievement. That's another important quality of a good guide . . . make sure everybody feels good with their accomplishments at whatever level they're at. There's no human dignity in degrading anybody's partial, temporary achievement.

Life is temporary. Life potential is only partially realized. We never reach our full potential. It's impossible . . . in my opinion. Every time I've eaten a piece of crap food, I've degraded my lifetime potential . . . a teeny, tiny bit. All of us eat some sort of crap sometime in our life. I know I have . . . and it wasn't always food or my stomach that was eating the crap. Some of the crap was digested in my brain. It's a journey, not a destination. In sports, in commercial transactions, in neighbor relations, in life, I believe all of human interaction can be beneficial if we seek balance and consensus.

Life is balanced if we seek balance. The universe is not some galactic zero sum game fighting against us in some epic struggle of competition. We humans create our own galactic competitive struggles. Collectively for sure, not so much individually, but sometimes we can work ourselves into a quandary of our own doing. I know I have. Life is abundant because the universe is abundant. I believe it's man's contrivances, his artifices and conceits that put that balance equation out of kilter and into a wobble from time to time in the cycles of humanity. We certainly see that societal wobble today in triple full house spades. Endless warfare and welfare tend to do that . . . put a wobble into humanity. We're wobbling a bit these days, in my opinion.

Summiting is not the ultimate objective of pure alpinism in my climbing manual for success. The process of personal alpine discovery is the objective. This personal discovery is far more valuable than the summit. We all have limits. Mountaineering has shown me that humbling principle. All of us have limits: Even kryptonite Twight, Shackleton, Tiger, and Einstein. We all do. Shackleton died at age 47 of a heart attack. My Business partner and mentor in the vitamin business, the capitalist with all the investment money, died at age 62. Cancer.

Last time I saw him alive was on June 17, 1997 in his house while we talked quietly. He knew he was in big trouble, but neither he nor anybody else had a clue of the what, or the why. That's why I flew down to see him. He called me to come and talk privately. We visited quietly for a while and he wished me god speed in my life. He knew he was running out of timber. I found it disconcerting to accept his failing condition. The very best of modern medicine in Southern California hadn't yet diagnosed his deep malaise. They found out the day after I left his house. It was terminal.

Less than 60 days later I took my turn pitching the symbolic solitary shovel of dirt into his grave along with his son, his other partner and the Rabbi. We were sending him back home to a very peaceful place. That's how I felt that day. He was moving on to a peaceful place. I'm thankful I could help put him to rest. I miss him. I think of him often.

Together with the family and the Rabbi, we broke bread at the Shiva. It was a beautiful gathering. That was the end. I wish back then I would've known I was Jewish. I needed to be at the Shiva for closure with a man very close in my life. I'm thankful the family invited me. I didn't fully understand how unique and special my relationship was with that man . . . until I wrote this passage today. This is not a healing for me today . . . this is a quiet celebration at a deeper level than at that graveside and the Shiva. It's never too late to acknowledge and accept deeper truths. He made a profound difference in my life and I'm forever grateful.

That number 17 keeps showing up at the most important intersections in my life. It's the last time I saw him. I need to keep my eyes peeled for more 17s out there. But where to look?

Just Took A Few Minutes' Break From Rattling The Keyboard And Am Now Back

My wife who has read every single world of this manuscript probably five times over the past month, maybe more, brought this little bit of irony to my attention just as I completed the last paragraph above. She's read none of this chapter yet. She has no clue what I just wrote one paragraph above, 5 minutes ago.

She said, "Jim, did you ever add up the numbers of your own birthday?" I never gave it a thought in my life . . . 1952. Maybe there was a partial hidden clue somewhere in this birth year . . . but what?

This is really getting a bit too stretched out metaphysically for me, I thought. I'm 64 years old and I've never added up my own birth year numbers. Something is going on below the surface I thought, but what? She's the typesetter and proofreader of all these pages. I barely know the basics for the

Microsoft Word program. That's as far as I've progressed on a computer. Getting all these pages nice looking is her work, not mine. When she reads over these pages, there's very little unknown to her. No revelations, except for the recent December paternal emotional purge in late Chapter 12. This has been my life on these pages and she knows it intimately. She, just like me, probably wonders will this long-winded rabble ever be of any particular interest to anybody. Who knows.

Only voices from the wilderness in Chapter 14 will probably ever be the real truth of that speculation. People may buy an e-book like this if they have Lyme disease . . . but will it mean anything to them? It's from those voices of the wilderness that I'll learn that truth. Is there a crust of bread for somebody in this massive heap of words? I wonder.

The Chapter 14 *voices* could tell all . . . if anything. I hope somebody can contribute to that number 17 idea though. That to me is quite interesting how it keeps popping up. Like the year I was born: 1952 equals 1+9+5+2 = 17 for the first numerical reduction. Interesting the coincidence of that number. I was born a 17 on the first numerical reduction of my birth year. Particularly interesting to me, I learned about that coincidence the first day after my 64th birthday . . . I learn I'm a 17. It feels about like when I learned I'm Jewish. Wow, I'm thinking, that's pretty cool. I have a hunch that I'll speculate on later. This 17 just keeps showing up at specific intersections of my life of some importance. It feels like the lottery drum keeps spitting out the number 17 on a little white ball, but dumps it on the table with no message where to cash it in. I feel like after this very important birthday, at age 64, a life map will become clear that'll lead me to something important. I feel like this book writing is a beginning.

Today's keystroke flow feels like stiff cold peanut butter getting squeezed out of my fingers each time I press down a key . . . slow, heavy, laborious mental and physical connection to the keyboard and then processed onto the screen. I haven't any reluctance at the keyboard today, just difficulty transferring the ideas off the keyboard up onto the screen. This is not easy fluid writing today. My mind is not entirely sluggish, but two weeks rest from writing has slowed my brain down markedly. I usually get the whole chapter in one instant flash. An entire passage of fifteen to twenty pages can just appear in a lightning flash . . . but then can take a dozen hours over two or three days to pound out the keystrokes to catch up with my brain wave. That's how I usually write: One lightning flash followed by a day or two worth of typing. It's not like that today at all.

Today the thoughts crawl out slow, orderly. Almost like the words are oozing out of the keyboard one at a time from a chef's pastry dispenser. I got the flash today, but it was more like a hidden flash. It's like a shadow that's appeared in my mind, and I'm interpreting the owner's thoughts behind the shadow. This is different writing today. It's the first time like this in this 74-day process of writing.

I Feel Young

I feel young today and this is very significant. I don't feel like I'm close to a retirement age at 64 years, even though I retired from commercial activity over ten years ago. I feel youthful . . . but not physically youthful. It's weird . . . I feel expectant about a huge future . . . but what? I sure didn't feel very young 60 days ago. As any reader knows if they've plowed through this book from the beginning pages, I never felt older and more broken in my life 75 days ago. Ten months ago, I had occasional thoughts about my last will and testament. Let me try to explain further how I feel. It's not easy to express myself on a keyboard.

Please be patient, Dear Reader, I know where this narrative is going, it'll just take me a few pages to get to the point of all this. It does all tie in with holistic healing . . . I think.

This chapter is not about my birthday. This chapter is about a transition into a new world for me. I feel like an ancient mariner sailing out in the deeps of blue water, who after a lifetime of years out in a vast ocean, can finally get a sniff of sweet earthy green living land just over the horizon. I can definitely smell landfall is approaching after years in the open sea . . . today . . . the day after my birthday. I could smell it coming a few days before my birthday. I feel like I'm on course to a destination that I've been seeking for a lifetime. I feel like I've passed through a distinct veil separating age 63 from age 64.

The several days leading up to this 64th birthday were different for me. I told my wife exactly that. I told her I could feel this birthday coming. She knows about my birthdays because she plans them each year. This 64 was a big deal to me in a deeply private way. It felt very good that I was turning 64. I actually anticipated my birthday for the first time in my life. I could feel it coming on. I could feel something was going to happen on this birthday. I anticipated what it was and it did occur on my birthday when I got out of bed. I suspect that for many people, their birthday is a pretty big deal on a number of levels . . . depending on a person's age and social surrounding. But for me, birthdays have never been a big deal. Never. My wife knows that.

I spent so many birthdays, Christmases, New Years and other holidays in the bush, in logging camps, or in social isolation, that these types of traditional calendar punctuations were never of significance to me personally. I just learned to emotionally shut them out. Sitting in some non-descript logging town, in a cheap ratty hotel room with a bathroom down the hall during Christmas Week, waiting for camp to open back up after New Year's, is a pretty effective way to remain emotionally isolated. I was an experienced journeyman loner at that type of insular life in my logging days. February 2nd, was just another day, in some logging camp.

My wife has tried to brighten up my birthdays with interesting destinations. Fez, Morocco, with whirling Sufi Dancers and exotic Berber food eaten out of ancient clay Tajine cooking pots, was one of them. Fez is the real deal. It's a medieval Medina of Biblical-like antiquity but all still intact. It's a spectacular World Heritage Site of some note. People call it the ancient Athens of Africa. The Mecca of North Africa. It's the biggest city in the world with no cars, or anything motorized. Just donkeys and sandaled people jungled up in an exotic life, that's at least 1,000 years removed from today's modern world. Some people are born, raised and die in that Medina, a highly spiritual city, without ever leaving its perimeter walls. It's an ancient walled city that's not some tourist movie set. That Morocco trip ranks right up there with one of the most memorable events of my entire life. It was a wonderful birthday experience, but it was the spiritual event, not the actual day on the calendar that's so indelibly etched into my inner being. The Moroccan culture and the sublime spirituality of Fez, and not my birthday, are what I remember on February 2nd, six years ago. I remember our guide who accepted and embraced our deep respect for their culture and religion and their way of life, and who introduced us to some of the sublime interactions between their most sacred spiritual people and myself on that incredible February 2nd birthday night. I crossed through a veil into another world that night with the Sufis.

How many non-Muslim people know that a Quran is read from the very last page and from right to left, forward to the opening first page and ends in the lower left hand corner of that first page . . . which is the last word of the Quran? I didn't know this . . . before my birthday night in Fez.

How many people know what the very first character, written in Arabic script of the sacred Quran, of the very first word on that very last page, is interpreted to mean? Not literally, but symbolically, and spiritually. Confusing you think? . . . I know. I was too. I was totally in the dark about all these things Islamic, until our guide explained a few things about the Arabic culture and Islam, back to the days of Mohamed.

That first letter of cursive Arabic script is one of the most beautiful expressions in the entire universe that I have ever witnessed . . . not by reading it . . . but expressed to me by the sacred Sufi hand signs, hidden from the profane. I hadn't a clue what was actually happening at my birthday party that night until the next morning over breakfast in the hotel. Long after the event was over and we had all gone home to sleep and then re-awakened the very next day, did I fully understand that I had crossed their veil of secrecy into their world of deep spirituality. Only the very next day, when the Sufis were all gone, did the guide fully reveal what had actually happened to me that night before. The Sufis all knew instantly, because of how I conducted myself with their secret hand signs, that I hadn't a clue. I had crossed a spiritual veil into their world. But only for one brief night. I'm not one of them, but I did get a glimpse of their world on the night of my birthday. They knew I had crossed over, the guide knew I had crossed over. I knew I had crossed over.

I had never read the Quran, held a Quran, or had seen a Quran before that night . . . nor since. I have never studied Islam, or been in a mosque during prayer. I'm not Islamic. Not even close. I'm Jim, the ex-logger, who is tapping out keystrokes on a computer recalling his birthday in Fez, Morocco six years ago.

How many people know how to respond if these sacred hand symbols are flashed, by a Muslim Sufi, to another Sufi, and then to a non-Muslim like me during their sacred rituals? How many people know what these secret interactions mean? How many Muslims themselves know of these sacred interactions? It's the most beautiful heartfelt expression in the entire universe I've ever witnessed from one human being to another. Although I was part of it, but didn't know I was spontaneously participating . . . I could feel it big time. They knew I was part of them . . . they could also feel it big time . . . but yet, I knew not these sublime truths in those moments. It didn't matter, they could read my heart, I could read theirs and I became part of them that night . . . in a very small but significant way during my birthday in Fez. I crossed the veil into their secret spiritual world. Somehow, my heart must have been considered worthy to enter their secret world however brief it was. My wife is the only person along with the guide who'll ever know what took place, but it was a very, very special birthday the night we had dinner with the Fez-Sufis in Morocco.

Dear Reader, I needed to give you all this back-story and

decorative sketching to tell you how I felt when I woke up the early morning on my 64th birthday.

The first day of my 64th year, I felt like I passed through a veil into a new world. I felt like I did in Fez. I felt like I had crossed over some geographic line of demarcation . . . but a mental line, not a physical line. However, here is the big difference than Fez: Fez was fleeting. I left my heart in Fez, but I couldn't take that veil crossing back home with me. It wasn't mine to keep. It was mine to experience only very briefly, but it stayed in Fez. That night will always remain in Fez with the Sufis.

What I experienced on the first day of my 64th year when I woke up is as simple as this profound truth: My life has just begun. That's what I sensed as this Birthday approached. In the few days leading up to February 2nd, 2016, for the first time in my life, I could feel something was approaching.

That future arrived when I awoke at breaking dawn. I felt like my life had begun as I swung my legs out of bed and it won't be fleeting. It'll be permanent. That was my 64th birthday message when I woke up and wanted to document in this journal of discovery and healing and celebration.

Tajine (Wikipedia) and Fez, Morocco (Wikipedia)

Chapter 17: Stuck In Base Camp

Tuesday, February 09, 2016, 6:46 a.m.

Dear Reader, I have to lay low in my psychological base camp for a while. I'm not ready to climb this mountain. I'm feeling a bit vulnerable today with the floodwaters rising overnight in the river. My knee is not doing very well. This serious knee condition is testing my inner strength and my resolve. I'm not mentally well at all today. The knee hurts badly. I'm a bit discouraged, even though the rest of me seems to be doing exceptionally well considering where I began December 4th.

It's the bum knee that's holding me in the base camp of my life right now and I've got a problem outside.

The river is in full flood and a tree came down over the dam and is about to lodge against our mill and cause big troubles. If that tree gets stuck, it could cause a massive debris build up, and then create a logjam. In these rising waters, a logjam could flood our house. I'm watching the situation very closely. This could turn into a real jackpot mess pretty quickly.

We always keep our three ready bags packed for these types of conditions and my wife and our dog are ready to get out of here. This place is designed to take high water because it's a water mill and it hasn't flooded in 250 years since it was built . . . but it's not designed to take a logjam backed up against the walls that abut the river. That's the problem. I'm watching that tree on the dam very closely.

The *gendarmes* are cruising the neighborhood watching this place. It's on their watch list when floodwaters rise. This is the first time since 2009 that it's been this high.
Tuesday, February 09, 2016, p.m.

I know those Lyme spirochetes must be almost all killed off . . . although I suppose there could still be a few lurking in the deeps. I'll continue the Teasel for a full 90 days. That'll take me into the first week of March. With 20/20 hindsight, I realize that the Lyme maladies were by far the most important aspect of my health to get under control first. I think my body was probably entering a total systemic breakdown by late November. That was only two months ago.

I firmly believe that this main mission has been accomplished with the Lyme troubles and I'm very, very happy with the rapid and powerful recovery from so many debilitating conditions. From what I've read on the Internet, there are some absolute horror stories of people who wracked their bodies using traditional allopathic medicine to accomplish what I just went through, almost effortlessly in the last 60 days. The little challenging things I went through like a few mud pie sessions, some spasmodic bull bellowing, and a Christmas Eve day and night of bedridden delirium, all culminating with a big fat headache on Christmas Day are nothing compared to some of the non-conclusive and repetitive healing horror Lyme stories on the internet.

Considering how down-and-out I was, that's about the easiest healing and recovery from Lyme disease I could have ever asked. Wow!! I'm just beginning to recognize how lucky I was to get through all that in such a short period of time. Plus, the father-son cathartic purge out of the clear blue sky. Wow! It's just now starting to sink in . . . the enormity of the healing I went through in December. It's just truly sinking in these past few days. It feels like I'm waking up from a post-surgery anesthesia to appreciate that I had an exceptionally easy and successful health transformation.

I've read all about this healing stuff in Storl's Teasel book, and I did write about it, but it *actually* happened to me. I've experienced it firsthand. I wrote about this guy *Jim,* going through all this, but as it turns out, I'm that Jim person in the book. Weird perspective back then as I wrote some of those passages. It was almost like an out-of-body experience writing back in late December. Incredibly lucky I've been. I've turned a nasty rock pile of compromised health into something peaceful, vibrant and alive, using God's human design as my blueprint. I've gone through a major holistic healing. I now realize that.

Two Days With A Chain Saw On The River

Thursday, February 11, 2016, 10:38 a.m.

I'm rapidly gaining all kinds of fundamental strength back . . . plus quick reflex action, and overall body rhythm. That I know for sure after cutting up a submerged tree that got lodged in the river during some interesting flood conditions that slammed us this week.

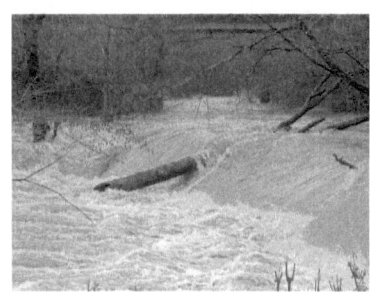 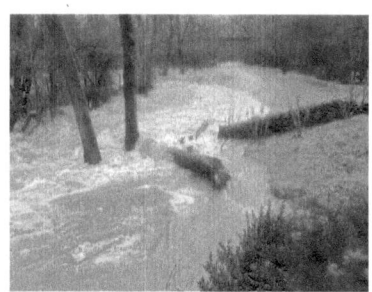

Winter Storm, February 09 -10, 2016

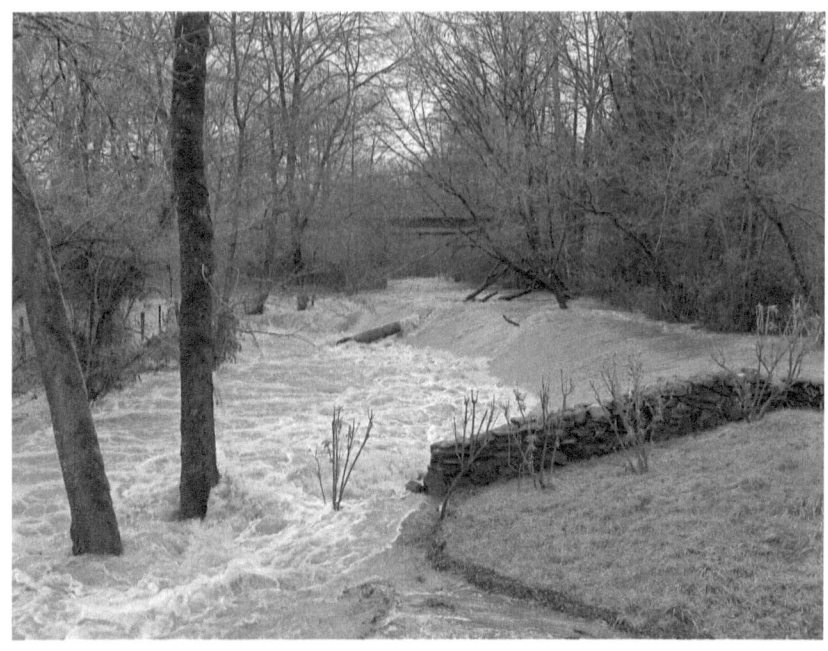

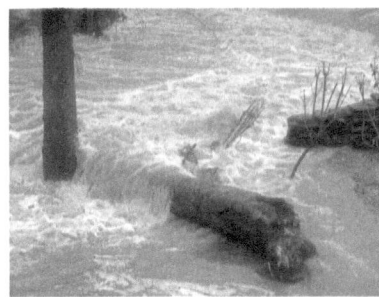
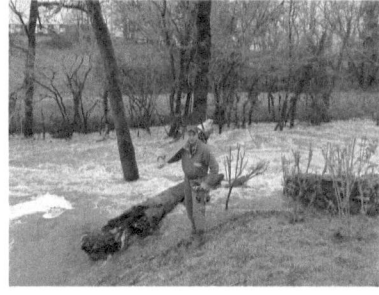

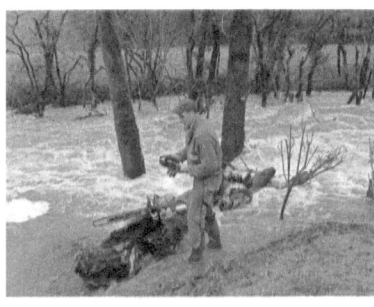
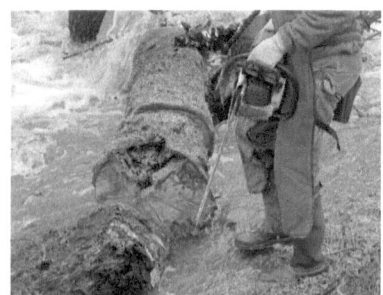

Winter Storm, February 09 -10, 2016

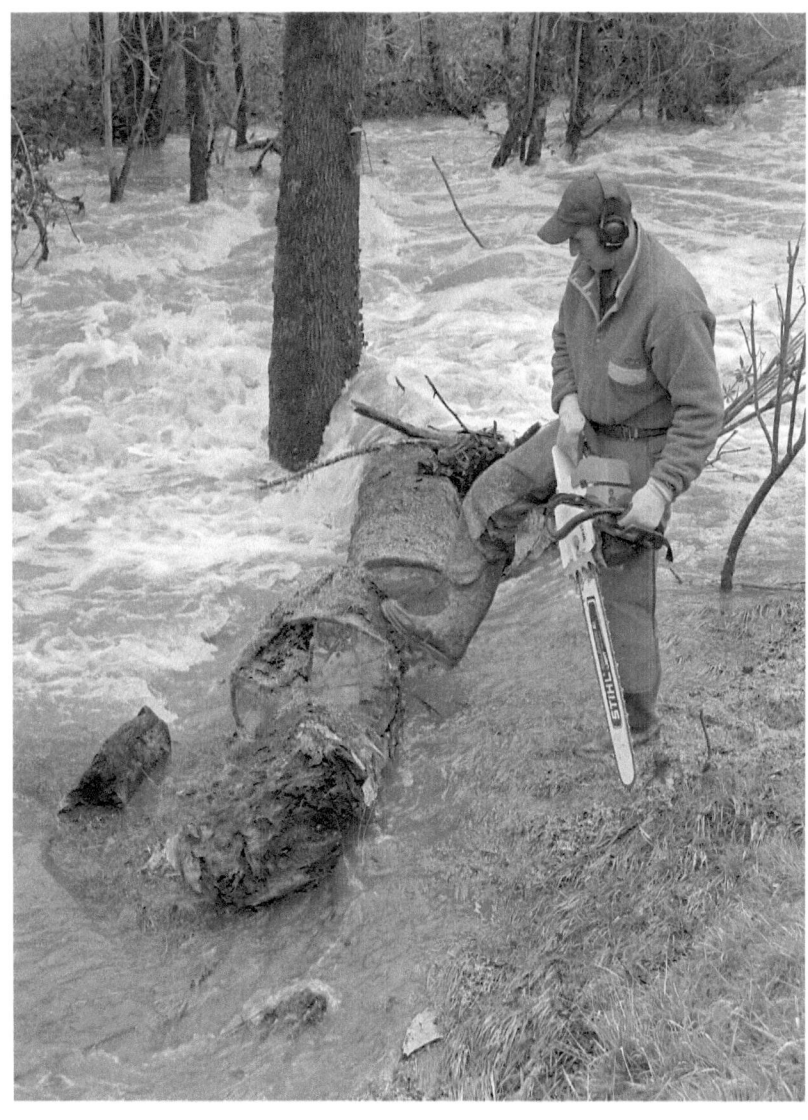

Winter Storm, February 09 -10, 2016

JIM LINDL

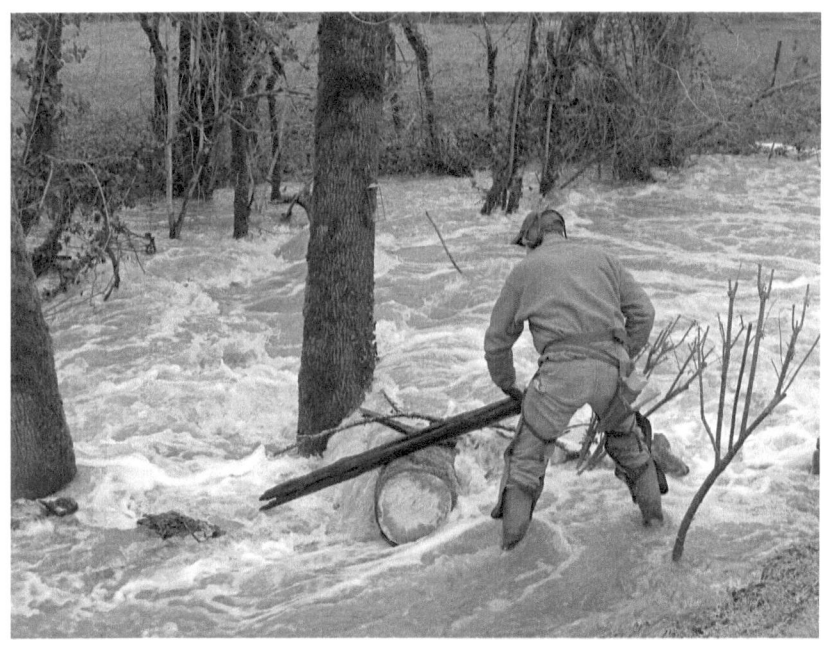

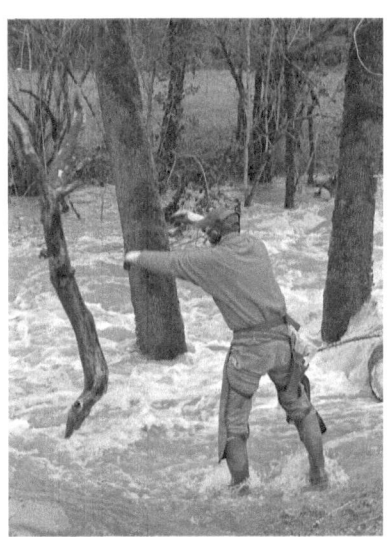
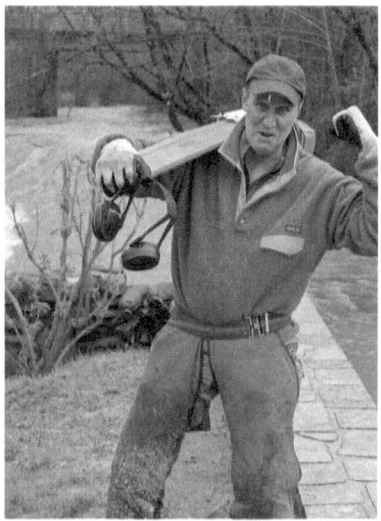

Winter Storm, February 09 -10, 2016

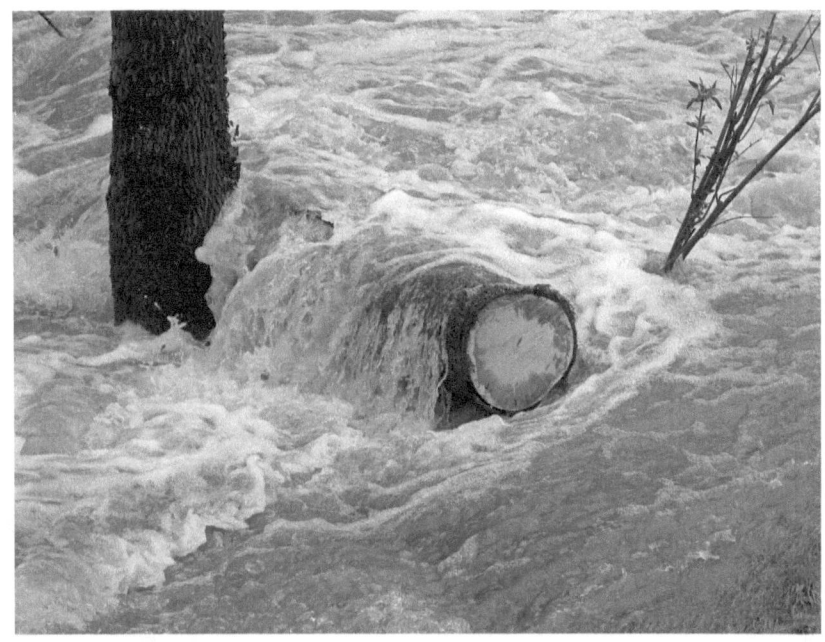

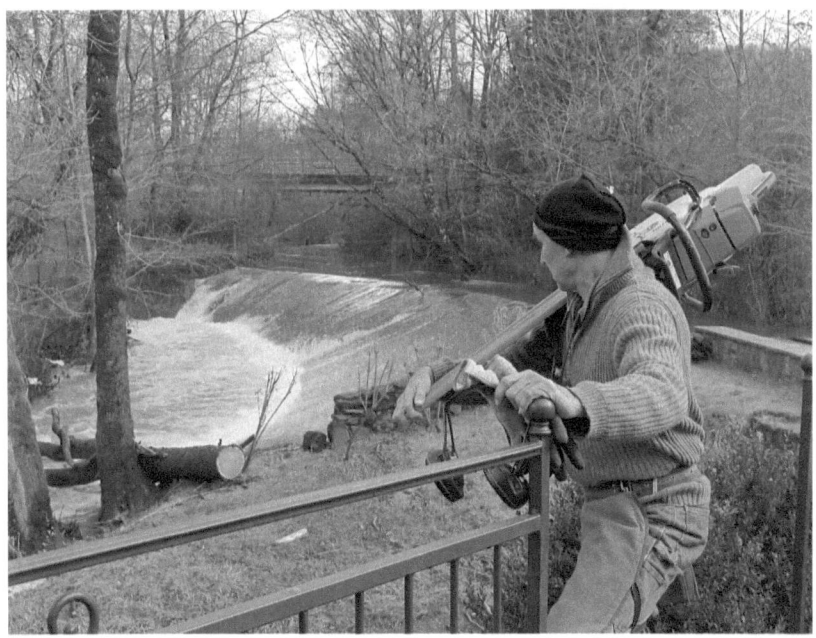

Winter Storm, February 09 -10, 2016

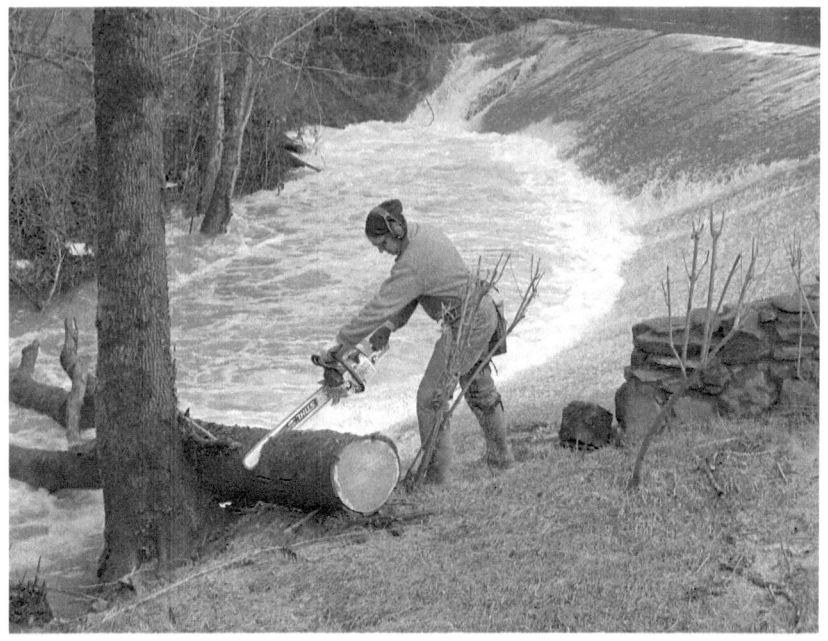

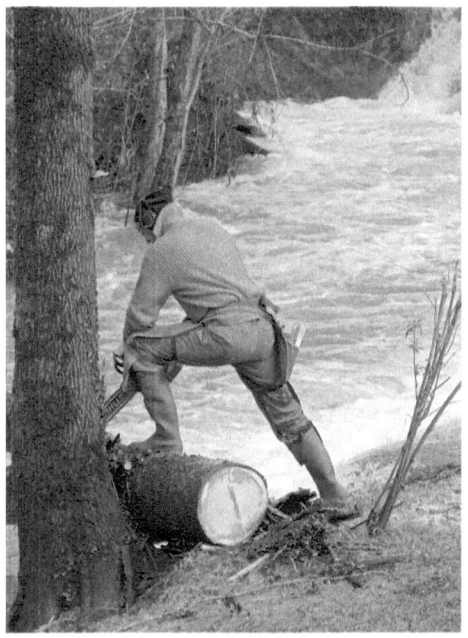

Winter Storm, February 09 -10, 2016

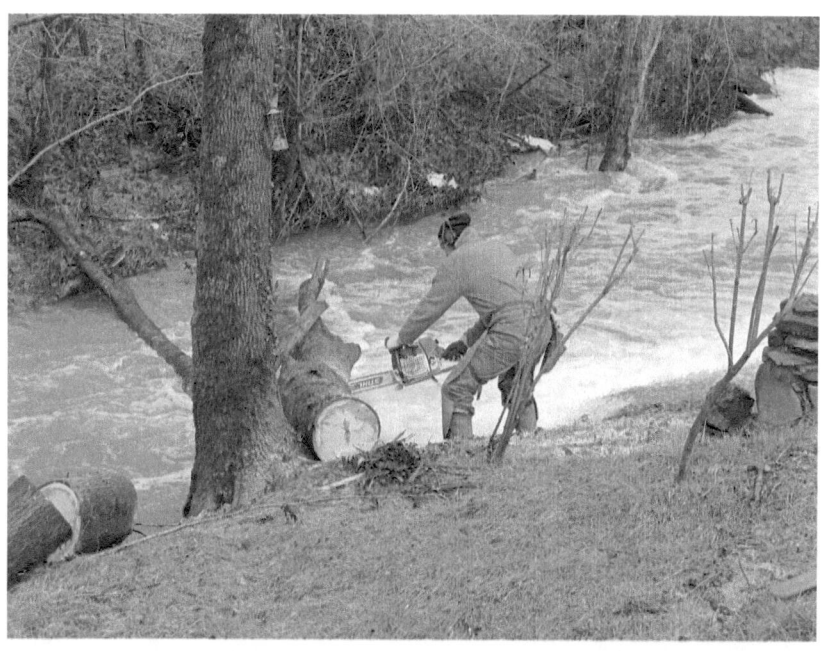

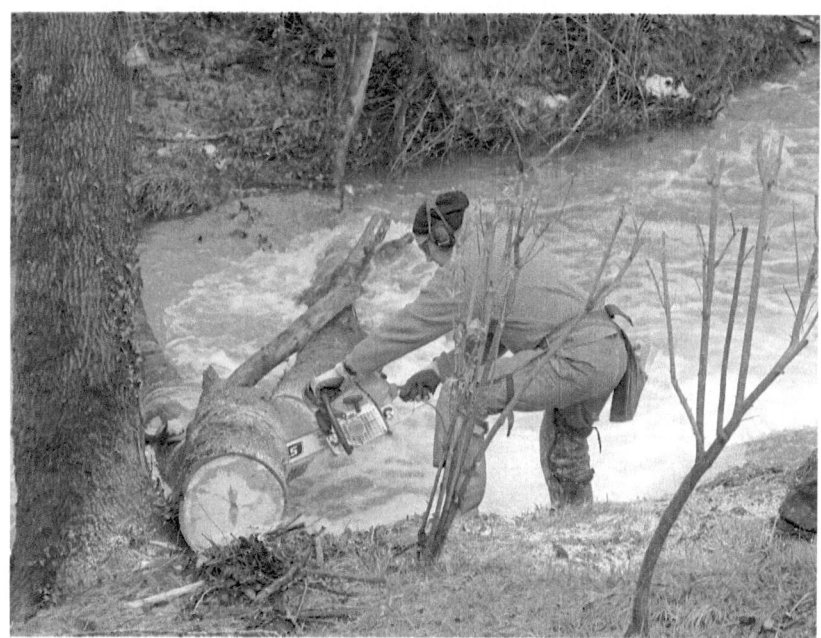

Winter Storm, February 09 -10, 2016

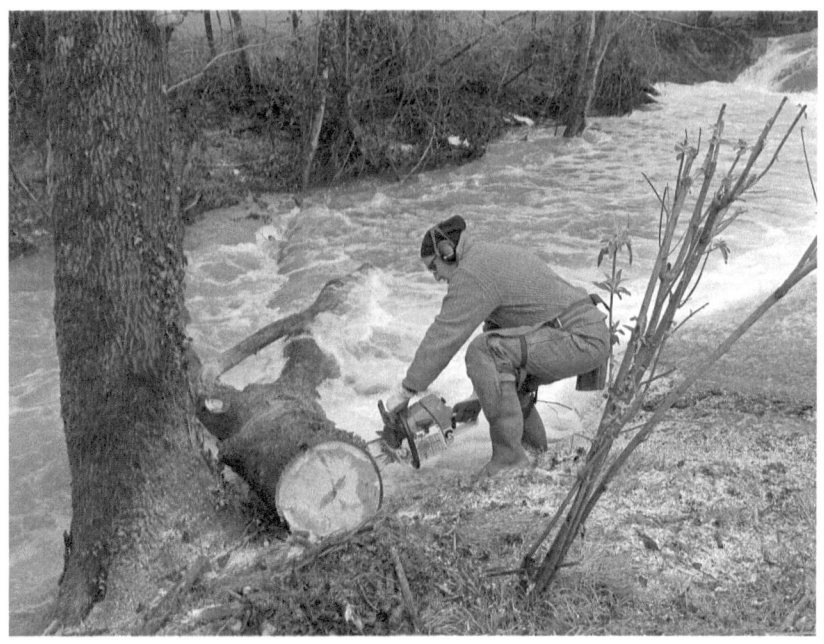

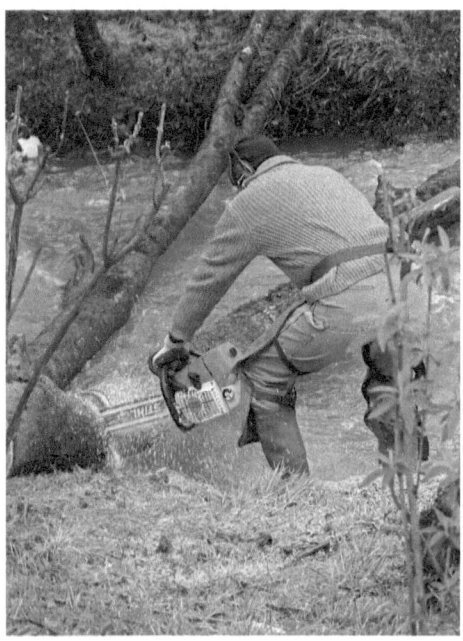

Winter Storm, February 09 -10, 2016

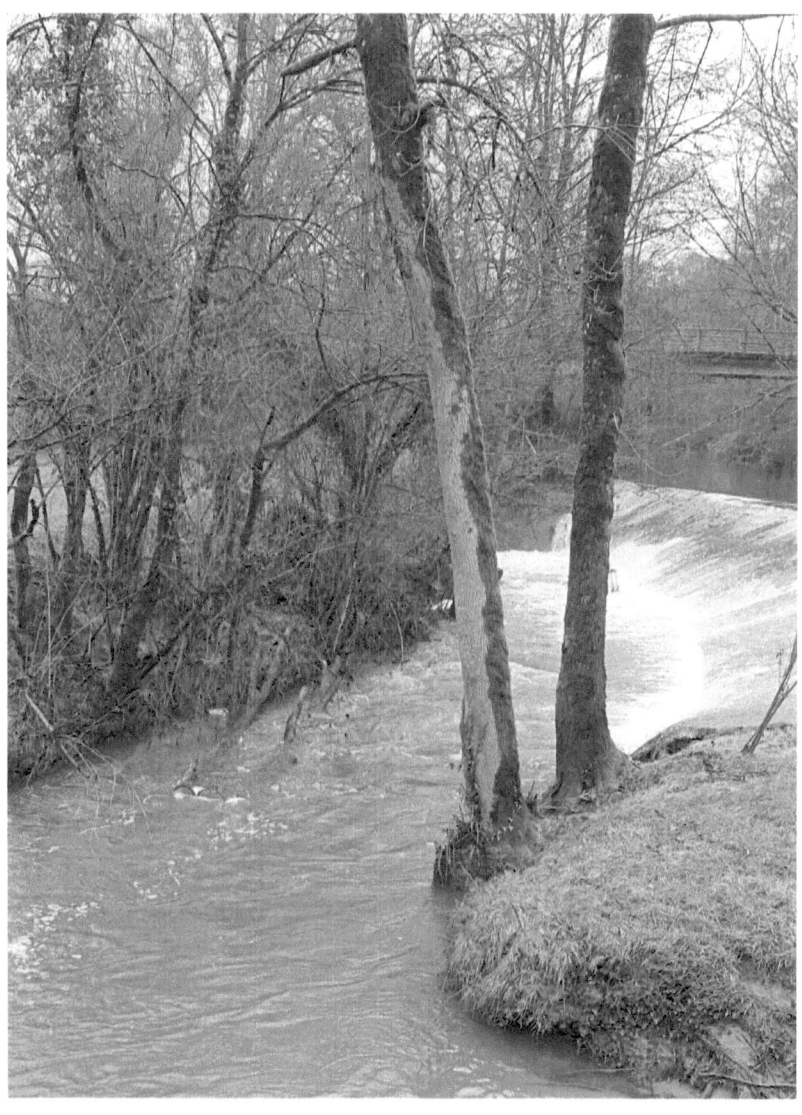

Winter Storm, February 09 -10, 2016

Dear Reader, this type of tree cleanup project has been my normal bailiwick for over 45 years. At least it was until about three years ago. Being an expert multi-dimensional logger, I'm keenly aware of the dangers inherent in handling a powerful professional saw, like the one in the pictures, in those swift water remedial conditions. That saw is two steps down from the very biggest saws, the massive production saws, used on old growth timber. That saw in the picture is not big, but it's very powerful and very fast. It can become instantly lethal with under-experienced hands on wet slippery ground and it can put an unaware person into a hospital helicopter faster that any hand-held tool on the planet. Statistically, there's no tool more dangerous than a screaming chain saw in inexperienced hands.

Sixty days ago, there was not the remotest possibility of me cutting up that tree. Particularly that tree, because of its position pinned across the river in the swift running floodwaters. That was a very dangerous situation for any saw operator. I've been hiring out that type of chainsaw work for the last several years simply because my reaction time and upper body strength, to safely handle that type of saw, in those kinds of dangerous conditions, would've been absolutely suicidal. I know the consequences of tiny errors in those conditions. Errors with a saw like that even in my professional hands, without the necessary strength, is a lethal combination. My mind would've thought I can do it, but if my body did not react correctly, what my mind wanted to do, could have got me a life-flight to Périgueux. That's why I've been hiring out chainsaw work . . . until today. I've known my limitations for the past few years.

During the past two days, I confidently and safely fired up that saw and made short work of what only a fit professional should tackle. I found it very easy work. I had laser-focused concentration on that saw blade like a PGA master with his putter on his final tournament stroke. It's remarkable how my whole muscular system, without any exercise in the past many months, has come back into reasonable condition to work a production saw professionally.

My knee is a whole other story. It's not doing very well. I cut that river tree safely because I knew how to position myself correctly out of harm's way. I was positioned so I didn't have to move quickly. My knee would not allow strong, sudden movements. I have a ton of healing to go before this knee is serviceable. I'm beginning to have some concerns. That's why I need to lay in at base camp and continue healing. My mind is as good as ever, and my upper body strength is pretty good considering that I've been inactive like a hermit for dozens of months on end. That chain saw work was a good test for me today. I'm convinced all my systemic muscle shutdown from the Lyme condition is totally gone. I could feel my lower back limber and free. I could swing that 23-pound saw smoothly and in safe positive control like I was out on the Canadian West Coast forty years ago.

If I had a good knee . . . I felt yesterday like I'd be ready to go back into the woods tomorrow. I know it's in me except for the knee. That STIHL saw turning 13,500 rpm's in that picture is a very familiar friend. It's an intimate mechanical companion. That saw for a few brief moments was an extension of my mind, through the arms . . . and into the hands to the throttle trigger . . . to the tip of that bar. From my back right big toe to the tip of that bar . . . I was one. I was one with that saw like forty years ago. It felt like I had a 2-cycle violin in my arms serenading the river with some finely tuned sweet music played by a master timber cutter of old. That was a very nice feeling for a few moments. I didn't feel old and broken while cutting that tree. I felt alive and useful again.

For two days, I was a Riverkeeper again. It's been awhile.

That safe, rhythmic fluid cutting motion, with that lethal chainsaw in compromised dangerous conditions, was a total impossibility for me only 60 days ago. I'm very thankful for my recovery to better health.

I'm healing, but I'm very concerned about my knee. I don't want to go through a surgery. I need to lay low and heal up. I felt happy after cutting up that tree . . . but I also felt depressed because of this e-mail linked below that I opened yesterday after finishing that tree. I'm not Jim Lindl, the logger at age 24. Not by ten million miles. My knee is the only thing holding me back. This is going to take some time to get my knee healed. It's not doing very well today and I'm a little bit depressed . . . but I do remain thankful and positive that I'll get out of base camp someday. I've not given up. I've been in way darker holes than this . . . only two months ago. I can't forget where I've come since December 4th, 2015. I hope all this makes sense one day. I'm going to go take a long nap and heal while I'm stuck in base camp. Knee Surgery Is A Risk Even . . . With The Best Surgeons (Regenexx)

Musings At The Water Mill In Dordogne

February 25, 2016, 6:38 a.m.

It's been two weeks since the river flooded. Everything quickly returned back to normal . . . which is normal. It will rise fast but settle down just as fast. The tree cutting pictures over those two days tell that story. This mill is only fifteen miles from the source. It's a small stream that flows both around and directly underneath this water mill and by late August . . . it's little more than knee deep. Just enough to keep all the visiting trout fishermen happy.

The *Cigognes* are all heading north again for their eight

month work season in the Polish, Lithuanian, and Ukrainian farm country. Flocks of them fill the sky day and night above our farm . . . all going north. Tens upon tens of thousands of magnificent giant birds flying in formation. They're migratory like Canada Geese . . . serious long range annual travelers. Beautiful giant birds which the English call cranes or storks. They build enormous multi-year stick-nest platforms clear across North Africa . . . all of Algeria, Tunisia, and Morocco. Their non-stop flight path takes them directly over our farm twice per year on route to cool northern farm country in February and then . . . back to sunny Africa in late November.

This annual migration cycle marks the beginning and end of the growing season at our little farm. These magnificent graceful birds are considered the farmers' best friend in those northern lands, and for good reason.

Everybody encourages their nesting on house chimneys, church roofs and power poles. These birds and the local human populations all co-exist across this northern belt of rich agriculture land quite happily during those eight months.

The *Cigognes* are an integral part of the farmers' non-chemical natural pest control in that vast northern region. They mutter softly when they fly. Beautiful creatures. Tens upon tens of thousands of feathered helpers are on their way north this month . . . like migrant workers . . . but free of charge to the farmer. No room and board asked or taken by the *Cigogne*. They quietly work with no complaints . . . no pay changes hands after a full season of hard work and they ask for absolutely nothing in return except a safe and clean environment to live in, and the freedom to raise their young and teach them their peaceful unique way of life.

They're not Muslim, or Jewish or Christian, or Hindu or Buddhists, or Atheists, or Anarchists, or Democrats, or

Republicans, or Libertarians. They're just birds . . . or are they?

Maybe they have their differences as well. I think we humans deep down . . . ultimately . . . all want no more than what these birds seek in life: Security of food, shelter and fashionable all season fancy weather apparel . . . a nice loving family life with a good apartment view across some fine country landscape or an urban cityscape if that's ones taste . . . mixed together with lots of fun, extended family to pitch in, in time of family needs and group security . . . unlimited freedom to pick the weather, and pick the time, and place of residence . . . lots of scenic travel with a nice four month winter sojourn in sunny climes. These migrant workers have a great healthy life, all tax free, without a myriad of laws and red tape as to when where and how they travel. Natural laws guide their behavior. Immutable laws, fair laws. Sort of like the Ten Commandments we humans have adopted. Equitable to all, understood by all and disputed by none for the last uncountable millennia. *Cigognes* are always assured a gainful dignified occupation in an essential farm service. Mothers are mothers, and fathers are fathers, and their offspring stay close in the region for their very long lifetimes.

Some of us humans struggle today to find even a smidgeon of the peace and contentment which *Cigognes* live so effortlessly. I think we all just want to be human and left alone in peace and harmony in our life with our family, with our own kin and our own kind. I wonder at the irony why we so dearly want peace and harmony, but it's getting further and further out of reach in the wider human circles these days? Is common mutual respect and common human decency . . . well . . . common? Or is it all fading to grey? Why do we struggle to find that perfect contentment like the *Cigognes*?

Can we humans ever find this Holy Grail called total balanced contentment?

I think about these things . . . all the time. It's part of who I am . . . and how I think and ponder since a very young age. My brother and I talked about some of these things before he left home. We talked about these kinds of things while plowing down Route 66 in that old Ford Falcon when I was 13 years old. I can't shake loose the stirring bafflement that these ponderings sometimes cause me deep inside. I carry them in my mind like I've carried a bad back for too many years. Maybe everybody just needs to drink some Magic Teasel and some Magic Mullein or some other secret herbal tinctures, and mutual respect will magically flow back into our lives for all fellow human beings . . . but I doubt it. I don't expect some secret convenient cure-all happy-herb will ever be found. I know there's a better way, a more peaceful harmonious way, but we're having a hard time finding that path . . . at least collectively these days. I firmly believe that warm human social harmony is hiding in plain sight, but it's up to us to find it, and let it flow into our life. It's up to us earthlings to let human harmony enter into our life like the unseen solar UV waves that invisibly flow into a flowering plant's leaves, and then re-radiate back out through its blossom into brilliant multi-colors of incredible natural splendor. I believe we humans are exactly the same . . . when a tiny little bit of human sunshine flows into us . . . we re-radiate that energy back with beaming brightness. That's the Prospector's secret. That's why everybody's drawn to him. That's why he can light up an entire room of people. He smiles a lot and listens a lot. He does it so effortlessly. I wish I was more like him. He's in the VA nursing home right now but I'm sure he's lit it up like a magnificent ball of colorful energy flowing out of his room . . . while he himself may be laying in agony. That's the Prospector.

I believe one of most incredible singular human to human wavelengths of magic energy . . . like magic sunlight that powers a flower . . . is the human smile. I believe that one simple smile, by a single person, at a pivotal moment in time, can re-radiate into a million beautiful feelings and things for a thousand years. I know this to be true. Smiles always multiply . . . until they're stopped in their tracks by a frown or a scowl or some cussy anger and bitterness. It's hard to smile at an angry person. I think sincere listening is the magic elixir that helps dowse down the fires in the angry ones. I know this to be true. A smile is so easy and free to give. Sincere listening time is just as easy to give. Two extra smiles per day by all humanity and five extra minutes listening to the angry ones . . . and I believe the entire world would change. I know it would, but there's a heap of unconscious long term daily smiles an precious minutes of listening needed to pull off that magic act.

I believe if we seek human harmony it will set us free . . . as free as the *Cigognes*. Smiling and laughing at ourselves just a little bit more might be a simple start. I also know there's masses of people down in the pit of despair and depression and funk and in an unfathomable bubbling cauldron of their malaise who simply can't smile. It's impossible for them . . . but not for us to smile . . . and listen to them. I know that will help, it always does. It's one of those immutable laws of nature. I should be so wise and compassionate to live these truths . . . but it doesn't happen often enough, because I'm so busy . . . with myself.

Dr. Emma Seppala PhD, talks about the power of smiling and the automatic multiplication of compassionate acts in this link. She's an engaging bright speaker and a noted expert on these matters. She also talks about the direct health benefits of social connection. Her wisdom is sought out by the biggest international corporations worldwide. Check out her biography. Pretty amazing Stanford University lady who speaks five languages. My TEDx Talk on Social Connection, Compassion & Happiness, by Dr. Emma Seppala PhD, May, 2013

I've learned in the past eight years from our incredibly prolific organic farm that garden chemicals are absolutely never necessary if nature's balance is sought. Garden imbalance begins when chemicals are introduced. Chemicals are not part of nature. Nature looks after everything perfectly if we give it a chance . . . and because we too are part of perfect nature . . . we're also looked after perfectly . . . if we allow its perfection into our life. Like holistic healing as one important example. Maybe just maybe . . . a bit more holistic living with a few unexpected extra daily smiles thrown in for good measure, is all we need for a bit more human harmony and less global wobble. Who knows.

Nature is not in conflict with us . . . today we humans are often in terrible conflict with nature . . . and engaged in sometimes systemic mortal conflict among ourselves. E-coli showing up in fresh vegetables at restaurants indicate, to me, a terribly imbalanced food chain wobble. Something is terribly out of kilter with the philosophy behind that type of factory crop production .E-coli are supposed to stay in the septic system, not find its way to the salad bar. Why does this keep reoccurring every few years? Do we not learn? We all know the answer. The answer is . . . that we know the answer . . . but we fail to heed the solution and we fail do the right thing. The answer is hiding in plain sight . . . stop doing what's hurting ourselves. It's that very simple. Just stop shooting ourselves in the foot . . . but me first! Stop! In ten million years I wouldn't eat at a public salad bar in America today . . . but I would in Marrakech, Morocco. And I have. We all know some things are out of balance. We don't smile inside when we read about these wobbly things we're doing to ourselves.

Dear Reader, I never share these types of inner thoughts with anybody. This is just me in private, stirring to get out of this base camp. I'm not sure if I'll leave these lengthy passages in this book. There're just some of my inner most thoughts about our human condition. These thoughts are probably about three levels deep from my surface. I sure don't plan to organize some avant-garde hippy-dippy thought salon or an altruistic cosmic-guided think tank to rattle the mental cage of society with contrived esoterically stretched thinking like this. That's not the solution to anything, in my opinion. I'm not sure what the solution is or even if there's a solution. Certainly in my lifetime nothing will change much . . . but I do know one central immutable law of my personal condition I can go to work on myself . . . and thereby, change myself and my immediate surroundings . . . and that's exactly what I plan on doing . . . at age 64 and counting.

Where Is This Base Camp?

Dear Reader, base camp to me is a metaphor for a mental space, although it certainly can also have a physical location. To me, it's that mental space quietly secluded in the middle ground between where I've been, and were my future lies . . . beyond the here and now . . . and somewhere out there, but somewhere coming up pretty soon.

That's what base camp is for me . . . it's a special temporary middle ground that provides some quiet down time and a place to pause, to reflect, and to absorb from others who have gone before. It's a time to rewind my tapes and enjoy the full length reruns. It's a time to ask, "Why am I doing this climb in the first place? It's a time to ask, "Can I do this climb?" Is it in base camp that I'm supposed to determine if I'm ready, internally, for what lies ahead or . . . more importantly find out what's holding me back? I need to ask and have answered in my mind, "What do I need to do to move toward my inner desires?" Or . . . more importantly, what are my inner desires aside from the obvious near and present life I now live. I ponder these kinds of pivotal questions in base camp. This remote mental place is a safe place. It's a place to decide a lot of stuff. Nobody resides in my base camp but my mind . . . along with all the rest of mankind . . . plus the entire universe that surrounds us to the edge of eternity. I'm completely alone in this quiet place, but also completely surrounded . . . by everything . . . yes everything. We're never alone even if we think we're alone. I see them and feel them, but they do not see me while I'm in base camp.

I suppose a base camp location could literally be a lounge chair on a quiet back porch facing a nice small residential back fenced yard. Just a nice private little place to hang out quietly. If I still lived in California, for me, it might be a rented cozy tent trailer for a few days out in Joshua Tree watching the full arc of the sun scribe its path, horizon to horizon, while just sitting out in open air until the stars put me to sleep in an inky black night. In my mountaineering days . . . it was usually the mountains. Remote and quiet . . . pure, clean and simple with no outside influences to disturb a dive deeper into the truth.

A weekend at a funky friendly Buddhist enclave or a stone sober Catholic hermitage retreat could also be nice . . . I suppose. Outdoor full wide open fresh air is my special place, but it could be anywhere.

    Place is not important to me. Intention and focus is what's important, I believe. Our tiny village has a beautiful thousand year old stone and timber church that overlooks our valley only a half mile up the hill from this mill. Its doors are open 24/7 to all, but it's almost never occupied with even a single parishioner anymore. Including Sundays. Just a few tourists and local pigeons stop in for a rest these days. The French Revolution kicked the Church out of France in one fell swoop but yet . . . all their magnificent altars and exterior edifices remain. Thirty thousand of these beautiful churches in France. Most of them have more pigeons than parishioners. Some have been turned into museums, art centers and community hangouts. Every teeny, tiny, little village has a beautiful church built long ago. Our village has only 270 residents, yet our little church is nicer than some of the finest churches in world famous cities with a million people. Around here these churches were built to last forever. At least the buildings were, if not their empire. The altars and pews and the choir lofts will still be around if the Church ever makes a comeback in this part of the word. Marriages aren't legally recognized in France, even to this day . . . if done by a Priest in a church. It's law to get married by the Mayor now. Priests aren't legal authority in France anymore. It seems like most young people don't get traditionally married in France these days. The popular option today, is to strike up a common property contract so the children and their eventual family land inheritances are all carefully divided up in advance. Napoleon made sure the Church's grip on the land was extinguished a very long time ago. The peasants carved it all up into interesting dribs and drabs of small acreages and plots as soon as the Church was kicked out. A large part of French land in our region was owned by the religious ones before the revolution. Neapolitan did a pretty fair job of turning the table over in the middle of that grandiose poker game. The peasants scrambled and squabbled for all the chips that crashed onto the floor that eventually created the rural patchwork quilt we have today in old rural France. A prudent person needs to watch out for those revolutions, I say . . . or at least anticipate where the chips may fall if the social wobble gets a bit more serious.

My Jewish lineage knew about French wobbles. Their personal table-turn happened before the Napoleonic era. The Royalty and the religious ones were pretty effective with their power monopoly back in the day. Interesting history to me but not so much to the locals. They mostly are just busy today tending to their animals and their gardens and their families and their life on the land they got from the Royalty and the Church, thanks to Napoleon and his sword wielding crowd who swept down though Continental History. Back in the day, the locals literally put in a few buried stone markers here and there and probably said, "I'll take this plot, how about you taking that one over there by the stream," . . . and that's how all our neighbors came into their land rights over 200 years ago. Nobody has corner survey pins around here. None, anywhere.

When we bought this river front mill and farm, a nice valuable piece of property, the Mayor dropped in and we took a spade out in the field right were the 500 circuit is shown in this book's pictures, and we dug and we dug until we found some ancient buried stone markers from Napoleon's day . . .

or so the mayor said. He brought a local resident witness to the unearthed stones and then . . . they got reburied for some future owner. As soon as we found them, he decreed, "This is your property line between here and that big oak tree," and he and I together, then installed all our hundreds of fence posts, right in alignment with those buried ancient stones and a few ancient towering oak trees. Nobody will argue with the mayor or any other local farmers about property boundaries around here. Locals and strangers alike just agree where the boundaries all are and we all seem to get along without surveyors, and lawyers for land transactions. It's the old way. I suppose the *Cigognes* would approve of our practical domestic civility.

Only during funerals here in our tiny village, maybe two or three times per year . . . does our church fill full and usually right to the back pew. Funeral rituals seem to give some people one final shove toward some kind of spirituality if they lost it along the way. Our church is a beautiful tranquil place to feel the morning sunlight from the east as it flows right through the stain glass windows. The cold stone floors are so old that their center isle foot track is all worn into a smooth concave path right up to the alter. A lot of folks must have walked that line. It was probably their door way to salvation and heaven . . . or so they hoped.

It never feels like a church to me when I go up there to sometimes sit and ponder my lucky stars. It's a place where I occasionally wonder how I got to this station of life. It's all fairly obvious if I honestly probe just a few levels down the elevator shaft into my past. It's all very obvious for most parts of my life. But yet, other elements, have no rational explain except blind dumb luck . . . or spiritual guides. I believe in the latter pretty strongly, and so did Earnest Shackleton and

Adolf Bitterlich and a few others who have stared deep into the abyss and survived.

These past two weeks, in this quiet rural water mill in Old France, was a good time to ponder my knee and this healing journey and my future. It's been good for me to be stuck in a mental quietude with a sore knee for a few weeks stoking the daily fire and thinking. I've learned a lot and some of it will be expressed over the next few weeks on these pages and chapters to follow. I've assessed my condition and my capabilities and I know where I'm going . . . and how to get there. Today I'm pulling up stakes and moving up higher on the mountain. I'm done with this base camp. Everything is crystal clear. I'm ready to climb. It may be another five years before I visit this place again . . . maybe never . . . but I doubt it. I like the feeling of being all stretched out in a private mental lounge chair for a few days . . . every now and again. Let me explain what I've unearthed in my brain as I now begin the most exciting climb of my life . . . at age 64.

Joshua National Park
Joshua Tree National Park California (National Park Service)
The Farmers' Feathered Friends
Cigogne Blanche (Wikipedia)

Why I'm Ready To Climb

Dear Reader, my knee is not a problem. My knee is my knee. My problem is my attitude about my knee. My problem is about my expectations about my knee. I now understand how I got boxed in with some frustrated thinking about this bum knee over the past several weeks.

When I rolled my mental camera back a few steps these past two weeks, to get a good wide angle view point of my inner thinking, a good clear view of my inner feelings and fears and angst came into crystal clear focus. I had to pull back just a little bit to plumb the depths and find out . . . why was I getting all angst about this knee? What was actually going on in my head? One of my mentors over twenty years ago taught us that real truth is only discovered on the 26th question below the initial inquiry. Personal truth, real deep psychological personal truth, is usually buried at least several layers deep . . . and sometimes . . . a lot more than just several layers. Truth can truly be *subterranean in the cranium.* This thought Guru taught us that our ultimate truth can only be found after fully exhausting 26 successive introspective questions below the starting supposition that we wear on our mental exterior and present as our public self. 26 layers deep he taught us. I usually stall out on the third or fourth level below my shirtsleeve exterior facade. I'm not sure that anybody ever gets all the way down the elevator shaft into their very soul, 26 levels below the surface. Some of our pre-birth reality is pretty obscure stuff indeed, but it's there none-the-less, waiting for us to discover.

The Secret Life of the Unborn Child . . ., by Thomas R. Verny & John Kelly (goodreads.com)

Well Dear Reader, I didn't have to put on a toga, burn some incense and howl at the moon to find my truth these past two weeks. I just had to reread and ponder the first several pages of *Mr. Teasel* to unravel my problem. It was hiding in plain sight. Here's what was holding me back and causing my angst about more than just my knee. Below is the passage on page five that took me two weeks to discover and unravel the source of my inner angst about my knee that's not healing up very fast . . . which turns out is also not the real problem bothering me at all. My bum knee is my current focus oh yes, yes indeed . . . but it's not causing my boxed in feeling and close brushes with fleeting sparks of anger and smudges of minor depression . . . deep down in the elevator shaft.

Page 3/4 From MR.TEASEL My Hero

. . . Today is Saturday, November 21st, 2015 as I've begun to tap in these first few keystrokes. This may turn out to be a running daily event journal or maybe a full blown book as time progresses. Time will tell. The actual day that this writing will be finished or released I also don't know at this time. My future knee condition and the ongoing Lyme troubles will determine when, if ever it's published. It's impossible to predict. It depends on the healing mysteries of Naturopathy upon my debilitating cartilage and muscle problems infected by Lyme disease.

However, I guarantee this story will never leave this screen for the public to read if I have to go under the knife for my knee, or if my chronic fatigue continues unabated, or the constant "lightning flashes" behind my eyes persist and the unusual blood pressure spikes and heart palpitations and other symptoms of malady continue like they have for many months.

Why would the persistence of these troubling signs stop me from publishing this running journal of observations and notes? Well, because the working title above would be pure nonsense . . . and I don't plan on changing the subtitles or lying to the reader about what really happened. So in a very real sense, as I wrote this journal's working title today, and began this introductory passage, I'm optimistically predicting (hoping, dreaming) that a non-surgical knee repair and Lyme eradication will result from the healing direction I'm headed. I hope it works out for my sake as well as yours, and millions of other suffering people faced with arthritic induced knee surgery or the peculiar painful mysteries of Lyme disease.

A tall order to be sure so why this optimism? Because I've researched and adopted a promising naturopathic alternative course other than surgery for my knee and a non-pharmacological treatment for the Lyme maladies that I believe will work. I'll begin this combined course of healing in about two weeks.

If everything goes as I expect, then this recorded personal journey will be released and, I hope, will help become a change-maker for future thinking about modern day self-healing. That's my goal in writing this journal: To make a difference. . . .

Dear Reader, can you see or feel the root cause of my angst in this passage above? It's so totally obvious to me now. Can you see it? Can you feel it? It was knotting me viscerally these past few weeks because I was heavily conflicted with the Teasel's near miraculous results on my Lyme symptoms, on the one hand, and on the other hand, my knee is barely improving. This visceral lurking personal problem was obviously staring me straight in the face because I've read this passage in editing and proofing . . . at least 20 times . . . but yet, nothing consciously registered as the source of my conundrum until two days ago.

For me, the foment has been building for at least the past month. But particularly these past two weeks since I cut up that tree pinned across the river. My angst is what caused me to retreat to a mental base camp to plumb the deeps for my conflicted thinking.

Mental *balance* is a very easy thing for me to identify . . . as is mental *imbalance*. I don't think about balance/imbalance. Never. I'm always a sunny optimistic guy. Always have been, all my life, but I can also feel the gravitational pull of imbalance. I know if I'm out of physical, mental and spiritual harmony if I'm not smiling inside. For me it's that simple. If I'm not smiling inside, for an instant, that's an indicator of something. If it lasts longer than a few minutes, that's the start of a trend. If it lasts for some time, and it doesn't go away, that's a problem that needs attention. I don't believe we should carry a heartfelt frown inside for very long without trying to identify the root cause.

Any lingering mental frown that lurks within my being, which can very easily be tempered by occasional internal smiling, indicates to me, imbalance. I always feel these internal frowns, even if I pretend to be ignoring them. I think we all do. It's human. Part of base camp reflection for me . . . is to stop the seductive convenience of denial and dig down to the truth which may be a bit uncomfortable. Especially this frown business if it's lurking in the deeps.

I had to stop writing for more than a few days. I had to consider if I was going to continue this process of recording current thoughts and personal physical observations. I began to question if this book is but one gigantic personal exploration of trivial pursuit. I asked myself, "Why am I still recording these sometimes zany left-field brainwaves onto these pages? I began to think this book may never end if my knee doesn't heal up. I considered these possibilities.

I had a major resolution to ponder before the keyboard would rattle again. I was stuck in base camp just as much as if I was physically crippled and couldn't advance up a moderate mountain slope. That's exactly how I felt. Without my knee completely fixed, I promised to myself a personal trust that this book was never going to be published. I wrote as much on page four. Never being published meant not being able to *make a difference*. This is what became the source of my angst. *Not being able to make a difference*. This is what had me boxed in tight.

I've had a near miraculous healing from those nasty Lyme spirochetes in less than 90 days. My brain function is as good as ever. On my 64th birthday I knew I was ready to go conquer the world like I was 25 years old. This book contains important information that can help people battling Lyme disease who don't know where to turn next. I know that for a fact. I was one of them. This herbal Teasel Elixir is magic. I know that for a fact.

I know the Mullein tincture is a magic potion with what it's done for me . . . that four decades of Chiropractic care has never accomplished within my lower back. All of this information is tremendously valuable to somebody, and yet, because of my commitment when I began this journey . . . I promised to never publish a word on these pages unless I could chase that badminton birdie like I was 25 years old. That was the source of my angst. I felt boxed in from sharing this holistic truth I've discovered. It was page four that had me boxed in but I did not know why . . . until two days ago.

Dear Reader, I want to tell the world this story to help some people beat their Lyme disease like I did. But I felt boxed in and trapped because my knee is not coming along. I had to get out of my own way and ask myself, "How long do I sit on this personal Teasel story? How long do I sit on this personal Mullein discovery? How long do I keep this information from others to read? "Why would I do that? What's holding me back?" I thought.

I can walk . . . I can function . . . I've postponed my surgery, indefinitely I hope. I hope to grow some cartilage . . . someday. Does the current condition of my knee preclude me from passing on some wonderful personal discoveries in this lengthy journal? I think not. I just can't chase that stinking birdie today. So what!! Big deal!! I'm not afraid if they cut off my leg one day and put a piece of wood on the stump. I'll get around. Consider all those poor Afghanis funded in a proxy war during their country's Russian occupation. Untold numbers of innocent Afghanis civilians have no arms and legs from decades of war disaster. Most of them don't even have a decent piece of prosthetic-wood to hobble through the rest of their devastated life, yet most of them never complain. They manage to keep a sunny disposition through it all. I should aspire to be as strong with my piddling knee troubles.

10-Year War Disfigures A Nation And Its People . . . , LA Times, April 02, 1990

I know my brain works just fine today, almost better than ever. *I need to focus on what I do have, not what I don't have.* That was my message today before I began this long winded rabble. I'm very thankful and ready to climb.

I'm Calling For New X-Rays

I've decided to call for a new set of knee x-rays at the end of March. In my mind there was probably little chance of any cartilage regrowth while the knee was infected and swollen and eradicating those Lyme spirochetes during the month of December. But beginning early January, 2016, I believe there's been a wide open pathway to begin some cartilage healing as per my original supposition. It'll be 90 days of knee healing time at the end of March. That'll be a good time to get a definitive progress report on my knee. I'll continue to re-x-ray every three months for the balance of 2016 and those x-rays will all be put into this report, win or lose, as they occur in real time. I'm not going to change the subtitle of this book. I'll let the chips fall where they may. I've postponed surgery and can do the 500-yard circuit pretty well every day. I'm totally stickless wherever I walk. My subtle limp I've had for more than three years is almost totally gone. The sharp pain is minimal most days if I don't walk too much. That's big progress.

I've swept the dreaded Lyme spirochetes out of my body. I've lifted my spirits and know I can probably walk on this knee and function enough without ever having surgery, if I'm careful. I just won't be doing much activity on it for now. That stinking birdie can stay in its container along with the other three goose feathered projectiles until I'm good and ready to fire it over the net and chase it back and forth across the lawn.

I've decided to publish this book regardless of my knee outcome. I've come to terms with my knee condition. I'm mentally packed, pulled up the tent stakes, and got my boots on and heading out the door to continue the journey to the top of this mountain. This mountain has been looming square in front of my nose for over a month. I know it's a wonderful feeling up top because I've been there before. Dear Reader, I'm going to take you to the summit of this mountain with me, so we can share that view together.

Chapter 18:
Farewell Mr. Teasel

Monday, February 29, 2016, 9:15 a.m.

I take the Teasel no more. I'm done. I began the Teasel on Saturday, December 5th, 2015 and from that initial Saturday, every day for the following 82 days, I mixed approximately one tablespoon of this potent German herbal elixir in about four ounces of water and downed it . . . first thing every early morning. Usually accompanied by my little quiet ritual. The last Teasel tablespoon was taken Wednesday, February 24th. In those 82 days, a total of three 500ml bottles were consumed. The cost . . . about $350. I'll always remember this period of my life with great fondness. I do already, as I backtrack to some of the earliest passages. It's been a journey from the depths of confusion and physical debilitation with some mild anger at times . . . to a nice high plateau of life with a great view of the future at age 64.

Some of those days floated by like I was in another world . . . writing about dog farts and the bellowing bull out in the field. The rants and nattering about economic fairy dust and Caitlyn. I recently considered cutting that Caitlyn reference, a controversial transgender citizen. I didn't mean to verbally abuse anybody. That was not the point of my comments toward ignoring his current fashion trends on the covers of high fashion magazines. I've since learned more about the conflicted struggle that transgender human beings endure. It's difficult for them. I truly have a lot more compassion for what that poor man has endured since age five. My written passage tells more about my state of mind, than it does about his. That's why the passage remains. I want unvarnished reminders of my truth at the time I wrote this journal.

Some days when writing, it felt like I was swatting at imaginary buzzing flies. I'm glad I kept a close journal of my feelings during this process. These previous 318 pages could never be recreated if they were lost, because my feelings and experiences . . . at the time of writing . . . can never be recreated. During this brief period of my life I swept the Lyme bacteria out of my system . . . but there was so much more that happened . . . all of it unexpected.

These past 12 weeks has been a little bit like the experience I tried to describe about the Fez birthday party and the Sufis. I crossed a veiled curtain into the world of Teasel healing for a period of time . . . and it captured my heart in some untold ways. But I also know it's not a world one can hold onto permanently. Teasel healing is another world, but just a temporary world, while the experience lasts. Teasel root tincture in not some permanent crutch.

Teasel is a pathway up and out. I think all these herbal remedies work the same way. Mullein is not a daily crutch. Mullen is a pathway up and out of pain and muscular tightness. I'm convinced these living gifts from nature are not like some human concocted pharmaceuticals which are meant to be taken for the rest of one's life. These magic plants are simply meant to help us rebalance and get on with our life. In fact, I believe a component of these plants empowers our inner power, but they themselves are not the power, in and of itself. We humans have to ultimately provide our own power to heal, to thrive, and to move up the mountain to our next higher realm of living and being. We have to use our God given design for self-healing to activate these herbal tinctures. That's all they are in my mind, they're guides to lead our body to healing.

I'm beginning to think that these herbal tinctures are almost like quiet spiritual guides in a bottle, but I have no idea how they accomplish that feat. For small money, with neither a Guru to follow nor difficult books to study . . . Teasel tincture and some vitamins was not a bad deal for a 63 year old hard-nosed Canadian old growth timber cutter to take for a spin around the block for a few weeks

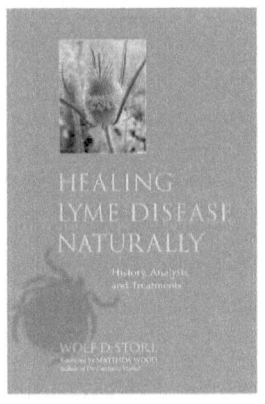

Healing Lyme Disease Naturally
History, Analysis and Treatments
by Dr. Wolf-Dieter Storl

Copyright © 2010 by Wolf D. Storl,
All Rights Reserved.

Final Lyme Symptoms Update

February 29, 2016

I have zero lightning flashes in my peripheral vision, which was probably the single biggest concern of the many troubling maladies stacked up against me back in December. No telling what was causing those brilliant eyeball fireworks, but I know they sure weren't a good sign. It must have had something to do with my brain or ocular nervous system. Those brilliant flashes would occur every minute of every day whenever I shook my head from side to side. I can't get my eyes to flash now . . . no matter how hard I shake or how dark the environment is when I try to raise a burst of lightning in my eyes.

In November, in broad sunny daylight, those flashes could overpower my peripheral vision as I walked in the garden. Just the simple foot-leg striking contact with the soil was enough to shake my head and fire off the lightning bolts in my head. I'm truly grateful they're all gone. It's now time to continue up the mountain. Goodbye Mr. Teasel. I hope somebody else finds you on this trail map I've left behind. It's now time for me to continue up the mountain. There's more to learn and more to explore. Goodbye Mr. Teasel . . . you're my hero.

A 100-Day Expedition To The Publishing Summit

Today is exactly 100 days since I began this journal on Saturday, November 21st. In 100 days from today, Tuesday, June 7th, I plan on releasing these pages to the world. This personal healing journey documented by this book, then incorporated into a self-publishing project, to me, has become my latter day Mount Waddington . . . a mountain I've dreamed of climbing since July, 1976.

The Waddington true summit is an icy fang that pierces straight up though some near impossible wilderness alpine approach conditions . . . and that's why so few have ever stood on its summit. In any given year, more people summit Mt. Everest in one single year, than have ever attempted to climb Waddington's true summit. Only six parties have achieved the true summit spire of Waddington in all its history. Achieving publication on Mr. Teasel on June 7th is my latter day Waddington. Let me outline the climbing route to this publishing summit.

My Waddington

Waddington is a highly desired alpinist prize. No, that's not correct. Waddington is an ethereal holy grail to some of the most elite climbers of the alpine world. Waddington is only dreamed about by mere climbing mortals. Only with spiritual guides is that mountain ever climbed. I know first-hand about this spirit business and I know it to be true about Waddington . . . at least through one man I knew very well.

It's one of the most desired sub 5,000 meter peaks in the world, and yet one of the most elusive to tens of thousands who have dreamed of summiting Waddington. I was one of those legitimate dreamers for many years. To summit that icy Waddington fang is so impossibly difficult, so elusive that only a mere handful has ever made it to the true summit. I was the roommate of one of those gods and when this project is completed, I'll tell you in intimate detail his scintillating account of the brutal 30-mile multi- week approach siege . . . and then his final 1,000 foot out-of-body ascent of that Waddington icy fang, as he told it to me, in the bunkhouse of a logging camp, forty years ago this August. Many Mountains To Climb:, Northwood Magazine, Dec 04, 2006

The Route to The Top

The check list of my eight pre-climb steps is simple . . . but will be difficult and elusive to fully execute by June 7th. It will be a test.

1) Get knee x-rays *early April* and publish in the last chapter of this book.
2) Continue writing and recording in this journal up to *mid-May* and consider that to be the temporary end point of this healing journey.
3) Continue to find pre-publishing readers to generate all manner of feedback on the book.
4) Probe the interest in the Lyme community about the information in this book.
5) Continue all possible healing approaches on my knee until fully functional someday beyond June 7th.
6) Begin building a robust and attractive website to eventually become the home and distribution nexus for this book and have it fully operational by June 7th.
7) Create a 501(c)(3) non-profit educational foundation that will own the rights to this book. This book will become the primary funding source for this educational foundation.
8) Identify several key founding members, who want to participate in planning, guiding and launching this project with me.

Now That I've Got A Work Plan, It's Time To Work The Plan!!!

The Teasel Foundation

Friday, March 04, 2016 8:00 a.m.
96 Days To The Teasel Book Launch

What are the future of this book and the future plans of Jim Lindl? "What's next?" you may be asking. This is some of the forward thinking that came to me shortly after I watched Dr. Glidden's optimistic lecture on Lyme disease and knee replacement back in October, 2015. These ideas have been simmering for months and now are coming to fruition two days after packing up at base camp. Let me explain.

Mr. Teasel has been pre-read at various stages of writing by a few trusted friends and a few people unknown to me. These first draft preliminary readings began after Chapter 14 was reasonably polished and typeset. This outsider reading began on January 24th. By late February, from those first few readers' comments on those first 14 chapters, I had an idea that this book would resonate with a variety of people. How many? The public would eventually decide that someday in the future . . . not me. But I was hopeful after these limited first readings of the first 14 chapters. I always knew the spine of the story (Holistic Healing) would be helpful to some people, providing my predilection to verbosity wouldn't overwhelm the reader before they plucked out something useful.

I don't know how many people will be attracted to this type of holistic healing journal and that will remain unknown until the actual book is introduced, in its entirety, to the public after June 7th. However I'm fairly certain the spine of this book is on the right track after those initial readings . . . and I'm grateful for their kindness to invest their hours of valuable time in a lengthy reading of a completely unknown book of questionable value. I'm grateful for their early encouraging comments. They truly put wind under my wings to move ahead with big thinking . . . dead ahead. I'm a promoter at heart. If I can help one or two with Lyme disease, why not one or two hundred thousand?

To me, although interesting as a challenging writing and publishing project, its ultimate value is *to make a difference* for other people. My Lyme symptoms are gone. I've solo summited that Lyme peak. Mission accomplished. The value of this book from the very beginning was predicated on *Mr. Teasel*'s usefulness to others. From the very first keystrokes I wanted this book to be more meaningful than just a decorative story about some ex-logger-guy with a bum knee and Lyme disease that was eating him alive. I didn't sit typing at this keyboard some mornings at 4 a.m. hoping to entertain people. I wanted to get a message out to people who may have been overlooking natural healing cures for their maladies. I knew if this healing program worked on me, I was going to dedicate myself to spreading a message of hope for holistic healthy living to other people, like myself, who had overlooked this important philosophy of health and healing. If my head had been stuck in the sand, I knew others were missing the boat too. I had set out to create a voice in the wilderness if this nutritional and herbal protocol was going to do me some good.

When I committed, and asked for guidance how to best create that voice, my answers came quickly as to how to spread the word. That all occurred within a few days of making the decision back in October to do "something positive." It was from the very first minutes after I was introduced to Glidden's first lecture I knew . . . somehow . . . I'd make a difference and that's when serendipity struck again. Within mere days after making that mental commitment to do something, I got invited, out of the blue, by a long, long ago and obscure business associate to review the process of *How To Write An E-book, by Pat Flynn*. It was from Pat's free 34-page PDF down load, titled, *How To Write An E-Book*, that the genesis of *Mr. Teasel* was spawned. I knew nothing about publishing any kind of book, about the format or the content of an e-book, until I received that Pat Flynn free download. That was the acorn seed. That was the very beginning of this book. I hope to meet Pat in person one day to thank him. I was inspired by his own journey and knew after reading his story, I could write something of value about my Lyme-Teasel journey. I knew that through a written journal of my own healing discovery, that I too could help others who might be stumbling in the dark looking for healing solutions. I just had to begin the process of pounding some keystrokes and I knew the rest would unfold if it was meant to be . . . and so this book came into being. Since November 21st, I've written, I've read and I've pondered every single day . . . at least 800 hours in total if not more. I now know this journey is just beginning.

This growing project is the product of an amazing wild plant called Teasel and a group of both silent and active participants. Some are direct contributors some indirect . . . some remotely involved, many yet to be involved. This Teasel Project is not about Jim Lindl. This project was just meant to be and I was the foot soldier who got Lyme disease and drank some magic German elixir and began tapping away on a keyboard for hours on end while pondering my future. I just happened to deliver the goods to get something started. That's how I felt as I was packing up at base camp just a few days ago. That's why I'm going to create The Teasel Foundation.

Getting Started
On Your Own Healing Journey

Sunday, March 6, 2016, 1:00 p.m.

It just occurred to me this morning that there's the possibility a reader may want to get started on their own program of self-healing.

Originally, my intention was to wait till the end of the

book to outline a few different options about getting started. I now realize this book has become a rather extended read, and there's plenty of good reason to get started . . . or at least get more information about the cost of some starter products and delivery details etc. Last week, several people with confirmed chronic Lyme disease, contacted me out of left field. One is from Ohio and two are from Georgia. So I know there's people out there who'll want to try the pathway I've chosen for the past three months. Those three people gave me the mental nudge that it's time to write this passage for new people unfamiliar with holistic solutions and Teasel in particular.

CK lives up in Billings, Montana and is definitely the one to get connected with for all things product related and here's why. We nicknamed her CK Teasel or just *CK* for short.

I retired a few years ago from the distribution side of the vitamin business and choose not to become directly re-involved for a variety of reasons that you'll read about later. I have definite plans going forward, namely promoting the general concept of *Holistic Healing Hiding in Plain Sight*. In other words, becoming more of a general activist to spread the word far and wide in a big way . . . and I do have some definite plans and experience about that type of advocacy once this book is published.

To be a good product dealer, it takes serious professional focus and dedication. It takes knowledge and superior listening skills. It takes integrity and commitment . . . to be a consistent effective help to customers. This type of personal business is conducted *one important person* at a time and . . . *every person is a very important person.* It's not an easy or simple business. CK has proven over the past 25 years that she's one of the rare ones who truly connects with people. Besides all that, she's a lot of fun to work with and customers love her humor. People enjoy working with her.

I've been closely associated with her in the high-tech supplement industry since 1991. We're longtime friends so it'll be natural that we communicate about any activity originating from readers of this book. I'll know what's going on and never be far away, even though I'm back in the shadows working on my own public promotion with the Foundation.

If significant general interest about product acquisition ever develops from readers of this book, I'll be ready to assist her. Quality product acquisition is also not easy, or cut and dried. If the ingredients specified on the label are not in the bottle, a person is not only wasting their money, but they're not going to get any results. Dear Reader, if you have confirmed Lyme disease or its nasty debilitating symptoms, that's not an option.

Until I'm convinced from personal herb farm and production lab visits and meetings with their owners, I personally will not recommend any herbal tincture at his time.

Europe, by far, has a deeper and longer track record in the exacting production of herbal tinctures. In general, I've seen, first hand, that Europe has a much greater consumer awareness and expectation about quality food grade, and that persnickety European awareness drives their entire system to a much higher level of excellence and expectations . . . from the farm field and the forest and the pasture, and then, all through the myriad of steps to the store shelves.

Only after consultation with world class herbalists like Storl, Wood and others, will I reference anything other than European sourced phyto-therapeutics, tinctures and all things herbal that we put into our mouth for anything more important than some tea at a restaurant.

Before a person runs out and spends their hard earned money on any *nutritional supplement, or any herbal product*, they should review this sobering reference from New York State regulators about recent misconduct by some of the biggest names in America, selling their brand of supplements. The Attorney General of New York has had some stern words with them recently about ingredients totally missing from their bottles of potions and powders. Shocking findings actually and . . . publicly released February, 2015.

A.G. Schneiderman Asks Major Retailers To Halt Sales Of Certain Herbal Supplements . . . , New York State Office Of The Attorney General, Press Release, Feb.03, 2015

I was an Executive Director for two decades in this industry and am intimately aware what goes on behind the scenes in food grade nutritional supplement formulation, manufacture and distribution. With Asian sourcing today, it's even more difficult than back in my day in the industry. Buyer beware . . . and know your supplier like your life depended upon it. I know mine did, just 100 days ago.

Product distribution and close customer contact is CK's bailiwick. It used to be mine too, but not today. I simply don't have the time to be effective for all the involvement it takes for good customer service. CK has the time and the desire to do what she's very good at . . . helping people improve their health with nutritional products . . . just like she did for me in October by finding the Teasel healing option when I seriously needed some help. CK is a problem solver and a communicator extraordinaire.

When I was in a Lyme disease jam-up, I sent out a May-Day signal to CK. She was the one who made a pivotal difference in my life by tracking down different people, which ultimately led me to Dr. Storl and his very important Teasel Book. The rest of this story and the healing all cascaded into my life from that point forward. I'm forever grateful to her. She can help you too, I'm sure.

I think it's time I broach this subject with her, before this book gets published so that I can help her get a system in place to smoothly handle any inflow of product inquires. I'm pretty keen on these European sources of herbal tinctures and teas, especially the German source of Teasel. I'm beginning to sense that this book could eventually generate some serious interest in Teasel's seductive healing potential.

Three people in the Lyme community are already in contact with me and they have more lined up when I'm ready to communicate the Teasel story with this book. I'll have to figure out an efficient connection for these European tincture sources back to America through CK and then on to the readers. I still harbor my old vitamin company philosophy: Whether it's two, ten or two hundred thousand, everybody's important . . . even if it's just one person.

This will be the last time I mention anything about product acquisition in this book.

CK will be ready for whoever shows up by the time this book gets published. There will be a link on The Teasel Foundation website to connect with her directly if people want to access some of the quality products I've been taking.

It's time to go to work. No more dilly dallying with rambling stories to soak up the time while I'm healing. I'm still healing my knee, but I've got an important appointment to build an educational foundation by June 7th, 2016 . . . The Teasel Foundation, with its own website. I'll begin the foundation with these preliminary philosophical guidelines of purpose and operation which will be displayed on The Teasel Foundation's *About Us* page.

The Teasel Foundation Founder, Jim Lindl, Believes These Principles To Be Important & Noteworthy

The Longest distance between two points . . . can be the short cut.

Vibrant health is the most valuable asset we will ever have.

People and relationships are more important than a gravestone that reads: "Herein lies the richest person in the graveyard." Especially when only a handful shows up for the funeral.

We should try to do all we can do every day.

We should try to do the best we can do every day.

The Teasel Foundation will always strive to under promise and over deliver useful interesting information, sound and simple actionable ideas from others, and provide community service without prejudice or preference. The Foundation's overarching objective is to facilitate outreach and connection with local micro-communities, to offer universally beneficial cross-cultural health ideas to help people live a better, more balanced, healthy and happy life.

As a non-profit educational portal, The Teasel Foundation website's mission is to raise personal awareness through a selected reading list of books, video lectures, and public discussion forums leading to Solutions Hiding in Plain Sight . . . . beginning with Lyme disease and undiagnosed Lyme disease symptoms.

Chapter 19:
Working The 8-Point Plan

Monday March 7, 2016, 9:20 a.m.

I t feels great to be motivated and goal oriented again. It's been a long time. It feels good to be organized, scheduled and forward looking and surrounded by a huge long term meaningful project that's under way. Writing this book now feels like only a very small piece of the overall puzzle while I was healing. The greater purpose of this book, I believe, was to get me back on track doing something that has a large social contribution. This 8-point work plan is my guide for the next three years. I'm now focused again, which has been my life long normal framework of living. Focused concentration is me. I can tell this is a part of the *new me* that I was feeling back on my 63/64 birthday transition. I've got something very meaningful back in my life and it feels really good. It feels right. I feel alive again.

Part of the 8-point plan is to continue my healing consciousness . . . and that will never end . . . because my changing health state is never static. Especially at my age, a person has less in their health reservoir account, and less ability to bounce back. I was pretty close to personal health bankruptcy only 110 days ago and I don't ever want to be there again due to benign personal neglect.

My grandmother was right: Our health is our single most valuable asset.

Once per week, on Mondays, will be the health state recording day in this journal going forward: Weekly observations, notations, and comments will be offered on these pages.

Regarding Lyme Bacteria

One of the critically important components besides the Teasel for eradicating my Lyme bacteria, I believe, was taking the Killer Biotic Capsules. When the Teasel chases those spirochetes out from hiding, something has to kill them off. That's the job of our natural immune system and additives like antibiotics or natural herbal killers. Killer Biotic, I believe, had a big role in eradicating my troubles. I took this herbal capsule product *daily for two months* and then stopped for all of February only to *restart in March*. I've been on it again for a week and will continue with it until mid-April. Why this interrupted pattern you may ask? Here's why.

It's my understanding that during long term usage of any herbal remedy, the efficacy of the tincture or tea or whatever means we are up-taking, the essence of the herb will diminish. Our body adjusts to the herb and its therapeutic effectiveness will diminish over time. So . . . the answer is to get off the product for a period of time and then restart. That's my thinking of what I did and . . . am now doing with the Killer Biotic. This product is a potent blend of phyto nutrients and also has a key component of honey bee production. There's something involved in beehive production that keeps out all unwanted bacteria from growing in the hive. That "special bee stuff" is also in the Killer Biotic and it attacks the unwanted nasty bugs in our bodies.

Your guess is as good as mine as to how to time these things . . . but for me, I felt my Lyme troubles were pretty well over by mid-January. If I stayed on the killer Biotic until the end of January everything should be killed off. I hoped . . . but!

One of the actual Lyme persons I've recently begun correspondence with in America, reports about his reoccurring troubles that just won't seem to permanently go away. He's been afflicted off and on since 2004. That was a wakeup call for me, and was my message to get back on the Killer Biotic for one more month. It's good timing because I've been off it for a full month. He's the first live person I've ever talked to who has Lyme. Everybody else, up to now, were unknown people. They were Internet stories of people out in the vast digital Internet wilderness. It feels wonderful to actually connect with a living kindred fellow Lyme traveler. We're both looking forward to sharing ideas and our notes about healing. That's what this *Mr. Teasel* book is supposed to do: Connect the dots for people seeking solutions.

Summary . . . Week 1: Back On The Killer Biotic

The rest of the Nutritional regime remains the same for my overall health and for knee repair.

A month from now I'm going to get another full knee x-ray to definitively find out what's happening with the cartilage. I suspect not much. I'm very much looking forward to seeing those new x-rays. X-rays don't lie.

These days my wife and I are busy figuring out how to use Wordpress to transform a stock website template into a robust communication platform for The Teasel Foundation which will eventually own, publish, promote and distribute this journal. Fascinating to me how all the brilliant computer industry minds with their vast technical creativity have come to bear in this digital age upon things like website building tools. Digital tools to me are almost totally foreign, except for this word processing program turning keyboard taps into ideas on a screen that will eventually reach people out in the digital wilderness.

My work with tools for over fifty years has been primarily mechanical tools. This is a steep learning curve, this digital world. This is truly my Waddington but I'm already on my way to the top. I can feel it happening with the feedback on the preliminary draft version of the book and my growing realization how many people are struggling with their Lyme battle.

Back On The Teasel Elixir For 30 More Days

Monday March 21, 2016 11:39 a.m.

Dear Reader, it's been two weeks since my last posting here and much to report. I'll get back to the Teasel/Lyme developments in a moment, but first I want to document all the development activity surrounding this June 7th book launch, website development, and nonprofit formation activity.

It occurred to me this week, that if my personal "Waddington Category" book launch project is successful, others who want to write their own e-book someday may glean a few ideas how they too can follow my footsteps should all this work. Soooo . . . besides this book being a primer on Teasel and Lyme, I feel confident enough in my business formations skills to know this discourse could become useful information on its own right . . . to somebody wanting to launch a nonprofit organization or an e- book of their own.

A Ring Side Seat To The Teasel Foundation Legal Work

Here is some of my thinking and an insider's view on how the Foundation and book got formed and launched in 100 days

I know the importance of striving for a good solid business foundation generally, but specifically before anything is launched. In my experience, cutting any corners up front in the formation phase, of anything, usually comes back to bite a person somewhere downstream. I like to say, "The longest distance between two points, can often be . . . the short cut." Shorts cuts in this beginning phase are not a good idea.

Good legal work and legal understanding is vital in this complicated world, in this litigious world we all live. Skimping on legal advice, and trying to save a few dollars up front can translate into enormous debilitating difficulties and costs down stream. Plus . . . going into a new venture of any consequence can cause a constant low level of angst for the leadership staff not knowing what potential dangers lurk in the dark. Everything from snarky tax auditors to frivolous lawsuits could show up one day and must be anticipated. Prevention is always the most effective cure

I was taught in business school that law can be used as both a sword and a shield. Best have both on board before launching this new non-profit, I say. I knew I wasn't going to troll the phone book for some cut rate one man band inexperienced lawyer to do any legal planning for this foundation. No, I wanted an experienced team bench for its depth and for its backup in all situations in planning and contingencies in the future. I wanted a team bench that's here today and will be here long after I'm departed . . . maybe a year from now, maybe forty years from now. I want them to have The Teasel Foundation's back covered.

Continuity of effective management and continuation of purpose is very important to me philosophically. I've personally witnessed the lack of basic fundamental forward planning totally wreck a beautiful, strong and vibrant financially bullet proof organization that didn't plan for succession and long term contingencies. It cost them everything in the end. Lack of forward planning ingloriously killed them off . . . stone cold dead in utter humiliating financial embarrassment. None of it was necessary with them, but unfortunately, inept planning in the formation phase sadly killed them off years later. The Teasel Foundation will not fall prey to naive neglect in the legal, financial or management succession arena.

I've selected the largest and oldest law firm in the High Plains States to represent The Teasel Foundation. I've found them easy to deal with, they're always telephone accessible direct to the attorneys on the project, every day of the week, and are eminently qualified. That's why I chose them.

For a few extra dollars, good council can make everybody's life less stressful and more productive. I want to encourage everybody's activity involved with this foundation to be happy, productive and optimistic. I want everybody to be creative and outward reaching and always focused on helping others find health solutions hiding in plain sight.

Crowley Fleck PLLP Attorneys

Building A Website With Global Outreach

It's patently obvious to me that a robust internet presence and implementing digital outreach across all social communication channels is a given for the goals and global scope of communication that The Teasel Foundation has planned. Lyme infected ticks live in the forests and the grasslands from Tasmania, Australia, 48 percent of the counties in America, parts of southern Canada, and certainly across all of Europe. And these ticks won't quit multiplying or biting. They're spreading and winning one bite at a time with no definitive cure in sight. The human population gets buried deeper and deeper with Lyme malaise each passing year. The problem of Lyme is not going to go away in my lifetime. This paragraph above describes the scope, the reach and the duration expected for The Foundation's education and outreach.

If you don't believe that longevity statement, and believe that all it takes is more money, and pharmacology and more doctors thrown at the Lyme problem . . . well think again. I don't believe that more money is going to help in the immediate term. It certainly hasn't helped much in the recent past thirty years. Just listen to this 12 minute video clip of an extremely well connected and famous actress that threw everything but the kitchen sink at her Lyme symptoms, and still came up short looking for a lasting and complete solution. Her story, I believe, is the approximate state of the Lyme community today. Yolanda Foster's Experience With Lyme: LRA (YouTube)

Take a look at the government CDC distribution map of *registered* Lyme infected people. This is only the *registered population*. By their tabulations there are over 30,000 new cases of Lyme each year. Other learned guestimates suggest it's at least *ten times* that number because of under reporting and Lyme negative tests. Lyme Disease - Data & Statistics (CDC) and This New Map Shows Your Risk Of Catching Lyme

Disease (Phenomena, National Geographic)

My personal French blood tests initially indicated Lyme negative. These sophisticated 2008 tests said . . . *Jim doesn't have Lyme indicators enough to worry about . . . but it is maybe a good idea to get rechecked. Then seven years later, in 2015, a new test using exactly the same testing procedure indicated the same antibody count, but it now further stated that the current testing results doesn't mean those Lyme Spirochetes aren't hiding from the testing methods.* That's a paraphrase of what my blood work said in French.

Essentially the last test said I may very well have Lyme bacteria present, even though the antibodies are indicating a relatively low count. I'll be scheduling a third and final blood panel in about a month and a new knee x-ray in about two weeks.

Teasel In America?

The Teasel solution that I've used is not unknown or unproven in Europe or the United States. In fact, there's one pocket in the United States, horribly infected by Lyme, in one particular county in Wisconsin, using a similar Teasel tincture that I've taken. My protocol was just much stronger in daily Teasel dosage. I learned all this in just the last ten days through some sleuthing. This group apparently didn't supplement their daily diet with any high powered nutritionals or the Killer Biotic like I did. Just the Teasel. I'll find out more as I open up communication with them in the ensuing weeks. These are knowledgeable people with all things Lyme.

Unfortunately, beyond that one tiny group, in that thinly populated Northern Wisconsin County, I've found that in general, very few people in the United States know about the effectiveness of Teasel. Numerous people wheelchair handicapped, like I was, have totally kicked out their symptoms like me in that one particular Wisconsin county. Most of them did have a longer healing time than me, but were very successful none-the-less.

This Wisconsin group uses a much lower dosage of Teasel than what I took. My dosage level was suggested by Professor Storl and the German suppliers. Plus . . . I employed a very sophisticated full spectrum nutritional artillery barrage to massively nutrify my system and thereby enhance my immune system. I believe that nutritional blast was a very big part of my massive detox and rapid result in 82 days. The nutritionals could also partially explain the minimal Herxheimer reactions I experienced. I experienced just the one quasi-delirium feverish event during the two days of Christmas Eve and Christmas Day. That was the only bedridden down time I experienced of note in the entire 82 days.

Why doesn't everybody know about this very positive Lyme success county in the United States? Lack of outreach and communication I suppose. No internet presence? No global outreach like what The Teasel Foundation is planning? No seriously directed promotional focus? No central blogosphere leader? Probably all of the above.

I'm now in direct communication with the highly respected leader of this Teasel/Lyme group in Wisconsin and will be introducing them to the communication loop on our website and blog so the word can hear their voices from the wilderness. Once again . . . a solution hiding in plain sight . . . like a n*eedle in a haystack* and people not aware where that needle is located. Buried deep in old rural Wisconsin is the one place the Teasel needle is hiding . . . in plain sight and used by a lot of people up there in the past five years.

Ditto for Europe, and even Germany. There are some

isolated European pockets of Teasel understanding at this time but not many. No coordinated global outreach being done here in Europe either. There are no broad based communication platforms like The Teasel Foundation is currently building. Germany is definitely ahead of everywhere else that I've researched, but as far as knowing what Teasel does for Lyme . . . just barely ahead. They've only become active, in their local micro-areas about five years ago. We're also working with them to integrate their voice with The Teasel Foundation presence so they can tell the world what they're doing in Germany, Poland, France and Europe generally. They're the people that supply the pure, high quality mother tinctures that worked so effectively on me. I took their specifically prepared product from December 5th to February 24th to knock down my symptoms as extensively detailed in this book . . . concurrent with the total body nutrification protocol including the Killer Biotic that has the bee hive cleansing agent.

They provided me with the Teasel elixir and they produce only green root fresh plant tincture, just like what the Wisconsin people took that remedied their Lyme symptoms. Mother tinctures are a very distinctly prepared formula of Teasel. Not all Teasel is prepared this way with plants they grow with exacting and controlled harvesting procedures. Correct harvest timing, either wild or domestic teasel, is critical for effective teasel tincture preparation.

Children in this Wisconsin county also got terrific results. Lots of children . . . and they responded as good or even better than adults with Lyme symptoms. Teasel worked on most of these people in this micro-cluster . . . *not all of them* . . . but the majority of them. Will it work for you? Only you will know *after* trying it, like I did. None of us in the Lyme community can or will predict what the next person's results will be. But for a few hundred bucks? Is it worth trying? You, Dear Reader, will make that decision . . . neither me, nor anybody else.

I also think that because of the current industrial nature of so much table food today, intelligent comprehensive nutrification is also extremely important to boost a person's immune system during the kill off phase of the Lyme bacteria.

My wife and I are traveling to Germany in early May to talk with these Teasel producers about the future of *MR.TEASEL My Hero* and The Teasel Foundation We want to prepare them for a potential wave of American interest that I believe is coming in the months and years after this book is launched.

Soooo . . . , Dear Reader, you might be skeptically asking, how on this extremely time challenged, hyper-distracted/occupied and technically complicated green earth, is this ex logger, a 64 year old retied executive, gardening in Old Rural France with a limp and a sometimes sore knee going to accomplish this Waddington scale global outreach?

Very legitimate skepticism considering my technology fluency ended 16 years ago with a Motorola Flip Phone whose batteries went dead . . . at the beginning of my reclusive rural life in 2007, and has never been recharged since! That's exactly right. I've never owned a Smart Phone, held a Smart Phone, sent a text message or received a text message, and have not a clue how we will begin to connect a Mr. Teasel Blog Site and a full featured website to Twitter, Face Book, YouTube, LinkedIn and all the rest of social media to reach out to the Lyme community. But I plan on having all of this up and running like a precision engineered digital Swiss watch by June 7th. How you ask? Here's how. Here's the plan.

I'm an executive first and foremost in The Teasel Foundation project. I've experienced first-hand some fundamental business lessons over the years in several entrepreneurial endeavors, and other private projects, but particularly when building up our vitamin distribution empire from scratch 23 years ago when I knew equally as little about the nutritional supplement realm. Also, I learned about extreme stress tested executive management when my wife and I built our ultra-complicated private California estate home in nine months from the first shovel to ribbon cutting. Those two epic projects, one of long duration, one of short duration, were consummate exercises in planning, executive direction and leadership.

The answer, Dear Reader, for planning, initiating, executing and completing complicated projects is to find other highly experienced people who *do know* what to do. Then coordinate, guide and lead those people to the finish line.

This Monday morning, March 28, at 10 a.m. MDT, our three foundation trustees, which includes me, are meeting with expert internet communication people to map out exactly where we see The Teasel Foundation headed over the next ten years across the globe, and learn how we're going to elegantly finesse a pathway through 7 billion people via the Internet labyrinth to first reach, and then sift through this globe of people to connect with those who don't know much of anything about Teasel, but could benefit by what we know. We want to lead them to our haystack and show them the needle. That's what The Teasel Foundation is all about.

It's that simple in my mind. They're the experts, not me. Sounds easy, but this Holy Grail isn't at all easy . . . and to me is about like climbing Mt. Waddington. This is an epic scale climb in front of us: Worldwide global outreach to the Lyme community in multiple languages . . . in three years or less. That's my summit objective with The Teasel Foundation. That's my later day Mount Waddington. That, Dear Reader, is what was cooking in my head in base camp a month ago . . . global outreach to hundreds of Lyme microcommunities over the next three years across the entire globe.

Delusion Vs Vision . . . There's A Difference

Dear Reader, I'm also not delusional about the potential outcome of this grand plan. I certainly realize that if this book is a dud, if it doesn't connect to the reader with some kind of very valuable information or insight, this global outreach will not get much farther than the computer screen in front of me. This entire greater vision either lives or dies on the strength of value to a reader of *MR. TEASEL My Hero*. That's reality. That's true of a new restaurant or a new movie. If they're both a dud, they'll both end pretty quick. Patrons talk about something only if it's really good . . . or really bad. I'm very cognizant of that fact. Readers, with their public commentary, will make or break all these grand plans. No amount of hype or advertising or loud u-rah-rah can turn a sows ear into a silk purse.

But know this; I've lived my entire life in this *cliché*: *"You'll see me on the top with our team in fine form celebrating, or you'll see me exhausted on the route to the top from trying."*

I'm not suicidal, but at age 64, I'm giving it my all. I wouldn't be launching this very ambitious public project if I didn't have high confidence in the outcome. Why the confidence you ask? Very simple. Firstly, Teasel works and there's a lot of people looking for something that works better than their current plan. Secondly, a handful of trusted first draft readers have told me this book resonated with them on a number of important personal levels. That's a start, and a ray of guiding light that causes me to lead ahead to the summit with steel resolve. Those initial trusted readers' comments and the power of Teasel are my kryptonite fuel behind this project. We'll figure out all the minutia details on the route to the top. That's what pure alpinism is all about: Discovering a path to the top that others can follow. That discovery is made by a leader with a vision.

Start Simple & Grow

I figure if I can personally reach and connect with three people, *just three people,* who have nasty Lyme symptoms and want to try the Teasel and nutritional ideas like I did, then they can help me reach three more Lyme troubled people that they know. If we four joined in our effort together . . . and can just do just that much again, one time more . . . then why not build a scalable integrated communication system to reach four hundred thousand people? It'll become multiplication of something very simple, one person at a time.

First we need to learn how to effectively find and communicate with just one person. Then duplicate that process via our internet engine. My overarching executive directive to everybody on this project is to merge *all avenues of any high tech with high touch.* I don't believe high tech alone will win the day. People thrive on meaningful people contact . . . people respond well to human contact . . . and a person doesn't need to read Abraham Maslow to know that immutable fact.

The Teasel Foundation will have a humanistic personal

connection incorporated into its activities. One of those connections will be picnics. Yes, Dear Reader, fun picnics. Keep your eyes peeled on The Teasel Foundation Blog. Our Blog and our e-mail campaigns will keep everybody in the loop about The Teasel Foundation picnics. Our public forum will not be a faceless cold screen on the internet. Our public forum will be in person at The Teasel Foundation picnics.

Dear Reader, right about now, you must be thinking I'm going totally crazy on this Teasel tincture. Visionary yes, crazy I'm not. I did this very same thing from scratch 1993 to 1997 … picnics and picnic type gatherings everywhere across America. From Carolina Style Pig Pickin's to big tent picnics in California to Yellowstone River BBQ's with blazing gravel bar bon fires into the inky black of Montana night. People like to talk to other people about their common interests in a natural open forum, without prejudices or judgment, or stress or pressure. People *need* to tell their own story and to be heard. People *want* to tell their own story and to be heard. Picnics are a terrific venue where that civilized cross cultural communication can exist in triple full house spades. I know this to be true. I've seen it, and I've done it myself all across America during four of the best years of my entire life.

Frisbees Vs Glock 9's

We began in April of 1993, with only four people, plus me. We began with a vision and a purpose to spread our message. By the end of 48 months there were 15,000 of us active *picnickers* who had an extraordinarily uncommon bond. Healthy living though better nutrition was our common thread. That's what we were all about.

People like to eat pot luck and get together and talk.

People at Teasel picnics will most likely be bringing more Frisbees than Glock 9's. It's possible. We did it in triple full house spades and people still fondly talk about it to this day. People enjoy the human connection of picnics on nice sunny days running into sundown with kids and dogs and extended family and friends and neighbors. It's universal. It's human. These picnics will be the human forums of The Teasel Foundation.

Back To Building A Website

The trick in web design is to find the technically capable and artful ensemble of experts that can help us accomplish this yeoman's communication network building task. I believe we've found a good match of climbing team members to get us started. We'll find out soon enough. I've scoured North America looking for somebody that resonates with our purpose and as it turns out, they were hiding in downtown Billings, Montana. The last place I ever though to look! It's at this meeting that a team of highly experienced and eager web builders, social media experts, graphic designers and copy writers will explain how they will help us accomplish these lofty goals I've set out before them. We will see. Building any website looks easy on paper, but getting it to function with its intended purpose is not easy. Getting our Foundation site to perform like I expect is going to demand something more than average dedication and focus by the designers. I won't stop until we find them. I don't know exactly how we'll get there, but I'll know when we've arrived. It will just feel right. It will probably take a few design iterations and many months of heavy operational experience to get it right.

    This is Friday March 25, 2016 at 5:29 p.m. as I finish this

passage. Monday, I'll report back to this journal with ongoing progress of my knee, and The Teasel Foundation.

It's Time For A Nice Glass Of Bordeaux And To Shut Down This Keyboard For The Weekend.

Monday, March 28, 2016
Weekly Update

Much to report, but first I'd like to post this link for the English/German/ English translation for teaspoon and tablespoon conversion equivalency. German Cooking Abbreviations (DanT's Grid Blog, Oracle Blogs)

The back of these German tincture bottles all specify the dosage in German and their notation and dosage routine can be a bit puzzling. I've corresponded with these Teasel Product Distributors in Germany directly to verify the correct interpretation on their bottle instructions. In the future, I'm going to request that they begin separate labeling instructions for North American customers.

A Teaspoon Equals 5ml. A Tablespoon Equals 15ml.

No problem if anybody expresses either the 5ml or the 15ml on their directions. But here's the rub . . .

What's An EL? Or A TL?

Dear Reader if you don't have a clue, join the zero fluency in German club.

EL is for Essoloffel, about 1 Tablespoon (Tbsp.) or 15ml.
TL is for Teeloffel, about 1 Teaspoon (Tsp.) or 5ml.
tgl is for Taeglich, daily

Furthermore, some of these German bottles specify a dosage like this:

1   Woche 3X tgl 1/4 EL
2-7   Woche 2x tgl 1/2 EL
Nach Wolf Dieter Storl   3X tgl 1 EL

Here is what this means to us English speakers:

Week One, Take 1/4 Tablespoon 3 Times Per Day.
Then . . .
Weeks 2-7, Take 1/2 Tablespoon, 2 Times Per Day

The last line, I believe, means Dr. Storl recommends taking it quite a bit heavier: One full Tablespoon, 3 times per day. That's a lot of Teasel and is 3 times heavier than the routine I followed for my 82 days to became symptom free.

When we visit them in May, I'll confirm all this labeling business. If you wind up ordering these products through CK, I suggest you might copy these translations and put them near your products for reference. I'm sure by then she'll have it all spelled out on her website.

Wednesday, March 30, 2016, 1:41 p.m.
70 Days To Book Launch. On June 7th

We've burned up 30 days since committing to the 100-day goal. Much progress to report on our march to the Waddington spire. It's been a well-used 30 days writing web content and planning the future. Measure three times and cut once I say. Planning is very important. We're busy with planning.

Cat's Claw & Sweet Wormwood Added For 30 days

I've not only restarted taking the Teasel for an additional 30 days, but four days ago also added in two more very important tinctures: Cat's Claw and Sweet Wormwood. Let me explain.

Professor Storl talks about these other two herbal agents as necessary to kill off the Lyme bacteria. According to him, and others, Teasel all by itself will not do the job effectively. My folksy explanation as rendered very early in this book . . . is that Mr. Teasel chases the spirochete bacteria out of deep hiding but something else kills them off. Namely our immune system or antibiotics or herbal additives that have the ability to kill off almost impossible to kill syphilitic-like bacteria.

In my case I used Killer Biotic herbal capsules and a very powerful nutritional routine to boost my immune system. Everything worked exceptionally well. Glidden doesn't offer any other alternative or additional herbal support so that's why I went with his suggestions at the time.

Back in late November, during my hasty, desperate and very Lyme foggy brain state, I selectively scanned Dr. Storl's writing until I found any and all references to Teasel. After doing that foggy cursory reading, I knew Glidden was on track, but unfortunately Glidden only offered part of the total herbal picture. (T.E.A.M.)

I failed to pick up Professor Storl's clear directive to also add in Sweet Worm Wood, Cats Claw and another tea to do the kill job on the bacteria. And . . . I probably wasn't the only one, because I see that these German tincture vendors now offer a Complete *Tick Kit, which includes everything that Storl suggests in his book!* These Germans did have it available on their shelf all along, but I guess the public was overlooking these other very important components to Lyme bacteria eradication. They're now all packaged together in the "Tick Kit."

Soooo, I'm now taking the whole "Tick Kit" formula for the next 30 days and I love it. I can tell you that the white porcelain target is getting nicely spray painted a couple of times per day, and the gaseous tooting is back in full three part harmony. Something is definitely cooking in my intestinal plumbing. That all began only four days into the whole *tick kit* regime. It lasted for two days.

Plus, in the past two days, I enjoyed a very, very deep three hour power nap after lunch. I think my body is telling me, there's junk still in my system that needs to go . . . and I need some more healing time. I feel absolutely great. Other than my sometimes sore knee, I don't ever remember feeling this mentally sharp on an active 16 hour sustained basis day after day, after day . . . after day. I'm very thankful. Life is good at age 64. 70 days and counting to June 7th.

I'm going to recommend that CK highlights this "Tick Kit" on her website. If I had to start all over again, like I did on December 5th, no question . . . the *Tick Kit* is the way to go. It's about 245 bucks for everything, for a month's supply.

Business Summary

The Crowley Fleck Lawyers are busy with The Teasel Foundation set up work. That process is fully under control. Great People. Nice people. Montana people. Straight shooters they are. Montana *is the last great place!!*

The web builders and internet communication experts are cogitating with their team after our Monday meeting to draft a detailed proposal for a firm fixed price to get us up and running toward our eventual outreach expectations by June 7th. They were empathic that our time lines are doable. That's one of the potential bottle necks that I see at this point. Programming and Beta testing is usually slower and more problematic than ever anticipated. Our site is simple enough, but the moving parts for e-commerce to sell the book and our learning curve to operate the site for overall good customer experience from pre-purchase browsing, to shopping cart efficiency, to post purchase communication and blogging, all the way to the finish line of them getting Teasel and other nutritional products into their hands and their potential to get their Lyme symptoms under control.

This overarching internet based process will likely employ E-junkie as a shopping cart service, PayPal as a card processor, and Aweber *or* possibly Infusionsoft as the e-mail communication and marketing campaign manager. Wordpress as the blog platform and Bluehost as the hosting service. Lulu, or somebody like them, will be eventually brought into the picture for those who want hard cover books. Plus a direct link to CK's website for product purchase. It's all doable but a yeoman's task in only 70 days and the programming has not begun yet! If this all works it will be a miracle because I'm the guy that doesn't even own a cell phone! For me . . . this is Waddington indeed.

Speaking of Waddington, I'm going to ring up the Q.C. Islands in Northern British Columbia today and see if I can shake out my old timber cutting partner, Adolf Bitterlich. I want to hear one more time, his final assent story of how, back in 1958, he mounted that *verglas* covered Waddington fang. I'd love to have him record that story, his first person account, as he told it to me in the bunkhouse in 1976. The clock's ticking; he's 82 years old this summer.

Teasel Bottleneck

An eventual bottleneck that I see will be a sufficient supply of the premium quality proven Teasel, FPTT (Fresh Plant Teasel Tincture), to meet demand. Much more exploration and discussion needs to be done in this arena before launch date. Teasel is a plant with a two year sprout to death growth cycle. The age of the harvested roots is critical. The roots must be harvested in very late fall and winter of year one, from a first year plant. After that, the roots are not any good. After this one year old green root harvest, it takes another specific period of time to brew up the alcohol tincture tonic in the correct ratios so it works effectively.

Making the very best teasel tincture is not unlike making fine wine in its exactness of process from planting, to harvest, to processing, to bottling. It's a labor of love and dedication to make the best formula. Very few do it all from seed, soil, sunshine and rain, root harvest and then tincture brewing to the bottle.

Some tincture producers use dried roots, stems and other questionable quality inputs and consequently the efficacy is not as consistently powerful as the correctly harvested and rendered mother tinctures of teasel. There isn't a lot of this premium product available anywhere worldwide, and not easily found on the market. Teasel production is pretty obscure today. That will have to eventually change. I want to keep The Teasel Foundation fully abreast of all the world's most exacting premium producers and our readers' interest in them.

There's plenty of opportunity for producers to substitute inferior raw ingredients, and yet . . . still label it as a bona fide Teasel tincture. The problem is, these inferior products may not work very well. In the worst case, a tincture producer may wind up utilizing two year old plants and roots. According to the herbalists' literature, a two year old root is virtually worthless, but the label could still call it Teasel tincture and not be misleading. The trick is to verify that the producer is in fact harvesting 100% one year old green roots and making their elixir from this most beneficial stage of the plant, in the correctly brewed ratios.

Dear Reader, if you think this is unwarranted scare mongering, think again. This is the modern era of bottom line corporate corner cutting to generate higher profits which drive stock prices higher . . . which can mean higher executive bonuses. If you didn't click onto this very important hyper link earlier, please do so now. It's about product malfeasance on a very disturbingly wide scale. A.G. Schneiderman Asks Major Retailers To Halt Sales Of Certain Herbal Supplements . . . New York State Office Of The Attorney General, Press Release, Feb.03, 2015

Just four months ago my life depended on a trustworthy supply of a product that I knew absolutely nothing about. Today I do know a bit more about Teasel, Teasel producers, herbal healing plants and European phyto-therapy generally. I want to, with the help of others, continually add on to that knowledge and to pass it on to the reader . . . through The Teasel Foundation so everybody is more informed.

What I do have in spades, is decades of significant experience dealing with people who own and run businesses . . . of all types. That's why my wife and I are going to Germany. If I can sit down for a long lunch and have an earnest business meeting with the owners of a company and their key personnel, in this industry, I'll *begin* to understand an enterprise's level of integrity. Moreover, I'll need to gain open physical access to audit their production steps from their field plantations and harvest methods, to process facilities, quality control procedures, and their downstream process through the bottling, warehousing and shipping steps.

In this due diligence process I hope to discern enough

about them as a potential suppler, to note them to the readers of this book. I want to know and trust the people I talk about in this book. It's that simple to me, but it's definitely not that easy. It takes time and close association to build trust. The Teasel Foundation will be around a long time. We'll always be on the lookout for the very best Teasel producers worldwide. I hope all of them contact the Foundation for eventual inclusion as a trusted supplier that the reader can contact for products.

These herbal tinctures have far too much importance to me, and I believe, to any end user to guess what's in the bottle if they're battling Lyme symptoms. Just because the labeling and a website may look nice doesn't guarantee the best possible product.

Good plants, good people and good process with an overarching philosophy of excellence, are the four threshold ingredients of a good end product . . . in my opinion.

That's why I want to visit with any Teasel producers before they get mentioned by the Foundation. That's why we're going to Germany. In the nutritional supplement company I helped found in 1993, this due diligence was standard procedure. CK is the same with her nutrition business for the past 25 years. She knows her different suppliers very well . . . or she doesn't deal with them.

Chapter 20: More X-Rays, More Blood Analysis

Wednesday, April 6, 2016 10:29 a.m.

A bit of reflection and some fun facts: The word Teasel is found 316 times in the book to this point, Lyme 312 times, Deep 115 times, and Dear Reader 57 times. I began writing this journal 137 days ago. Total word count to this word? 96,640.

103 days ago, Christmas day, 2015, I was in a very deep healing period and I had only been on the protocol for 20 days at that time. I sure wasn't thinking about global outreach, non-profit foundations or anything remotely related to chapter 19's big plans. Yet today, as I tap in these keystrokes, I feel like it's the best period of my life. Right now, right here, today. This has been an extraordinary personal transformation of feeling, thinking, attitude, confidence and belief in myself since December 5th. This is who I want to be. This is how I want to feel every day. That broken spirited Jim Lindl from last summer is gone. POOF!! Gone!!

It's 63 days to the planned book/website launch, on June 7th. Everything's in place. Everything's in motion. The Teasel Foundation, a Public Benefit Corporation, is now registered in the State of Montana. The 501(c)(3) IRS status is being advanced by the lawyers.

The web builders are contracted and in intense focused full motion with their yeoman's task of everything web related. We have substantial pre written website content ready to upload to their programmers. Their team is in place and will begin Friday.

This Friday I have a doctor's appointment to get the lab prescriptions for new Lyme blood work and new knee x-rays.

My knee is much better with hardly any pain at all. My brain is firing on all eight cylinders and operating effectively on high octane full power. My wife is handling all the paper flow and back office details. CK is gearing up for her supply company's linkage with Mr. Teasel readers.

The German Teasel Producers Are Waiting For Our Visit In Early May.

That's the summary of our current state of affairs in our planned 100-day march to the publishing summit. It's taken us 37 days of planning, study, writing and doing to get to this point. This activity we're doing now is called the "approach" to the summit in mountaineering parlance. Adolf Bitterlich's "approach" to Waddington took him and his party weeks of extreme wilderness bushwhacking to get to that ultimate final pinnacle, that impossible icy fang. No roads, no trails, no helicopter support, no GPS, no nothing, except kryptonite determination. He didn't make it the first time. He was stopped 1,000 feet below the summit with impossible climbing conditions. Weeks upon grinding weeks of determined effort to get so close yet he was stopped only six rope lengths from his dream. He and his brother were beaten, but only temporarily. They had to go back to planning, make some adjustments and refine their strategies. They tried again a second time the following year. Skunked again. Same story . . . then more planning and more adjustments to team members. Then he tried again for his third attempt two years later. He finally made it the third time. He, in August, 1958, was the first Canadian to summit Waddington. Adolf publicly reported that he was walking on clouds that day. Someday I'll tell you the rest of his intimate story as told to me in that logging camp bunkhouse 40 years ago. The spirits were with him on that final 1000 foot climb. I was 24 years old . . . he was 42. We were both old growth timber cutters sharing our unique lives for a brief moment in time.

We have 63 days left and are on track as planned. I'm very thankful for everything and everybody connected to The Teasel Foundation. Very thankful. For some time now, I've felt that some benevolent force is looking kindly upon all this activity.

Monday, April 11, 2016, 9:19 a.m.

This whole project is coming into crystal clear focus. I clearly see how it's supposed to look and function by launch date, and then a year from now, and then maybe two or three more years from now. The trick is to pull it all together and begin the smooth, efficient operation of all these moving parts. This whole grand project would never be remotely possible without the many people involved in the different aspects of the design, development and implementation. I've always lived by the acronym:

T.E.A.M. Together, Everybody Achieves More.

Never a truer statement than in this Teasel Foundation project and book publishing.

Nothing new to report health wise, except that I started taking a very powerful L-Arginine complex product for my knee. I've been on it for five days. More details about it later. My knee is the laggard in this long healing journey.

One of the biggest problems with re-growing knee cartilage is that there's very little, if any, blood flow directly to the cartilage area, and without blood flow . . . growth is difficult, if not impossible. This particular product recommended by CK, has properties that clinically show how blood flow is greatly improved in certain tissue areas, particularly the heart muscle. My thinking is that if it can help blood flow to the heart, why not the cartilage area too? I'm getting both of my knees x-rayed this Tuesday so I'll have a definitive baseline to compare to going forward. I suspect there's been very little if any cartilage improvement in my right knee. That's how it feels after four months. The Lyme symptoms are totally gone but the knee is another ongoing healing story. Thankfully I've avoided surgery and can function okay . . . but just barely.

120 Kilos, 265 Pounds, 1.5 Kilometers, 4 Tons

Having said that about minimal knee function, the chronic knee pain is almost non-existent lately unless I stress that joint by over working it, like yesterday. It's spring time here on the farm and everything is growing, including the grass, and the flower beds, and the asparagus. That means it's time to fertilize the non-vegetable areas.

The following short narrative is a comparison to my physical condition on December 5th, just 128 days ago, when I could walk no more than 160 meters and barely lift a few half sacs of groceries out of the car. I crashed in mental and physical fatigue every day by 4 p.m. back then. It's a lot different today . . . a lot different.

Yesterday, Sunday, I hand spread 265 pounds of organic

granular fertilizer over the ornamental beds and lawn areas of our property. It's a very cut-up and convoluted river valley property with multiple fence lines, and numerous stone retaining walls. The residential portion of this farm has a beautiful mixture of hedges, flower beds and developed lawn areas with a mill pond, river frontage and mill raceways all in the mix. It's truly a gorgeous estate property . . . but it takes maintenance . . . a lot of rigorous manual labor and hand maintenance.

To spread that amount of fertilizer over this entire property is a significant walking exercise . . . about 1,500 meters. That's over a mile of walking. The fertilizer is spread by carrying an applicator rig worn with a neck/shoulder strap. Filled with fertilizer, this unit weighs about 30 pounds. It's carried and spun by hand cranking a flywheel to get the fertilizer cast out in all directions when a person walks about the terrain. Very effective tool for small areas less than five acres.

Yesterday I walked and carried that fertilizer rig until the entire 265 pounds was spread and everything was covered. Rain was coming in the evening and it needed to be done. That took four hours, from 2 to 6 p.m. Then I attacked my two prized compost piles. They're huge and have about 2 tons of compost in each one. Rich farm debris compost needs to be turned every once in a while and before a good soaking rain is an excellent time to stir the pot. Rain was on its way so it had to be turned.

Dear Reader, how does a person turn and mix 4 tons of wet compost? With a special type of walk behind Honda rototiller. That's how I do it.

From 6 to 7:30 p.m. yesterday evening I hand wrestled and crisscrossed that rototiller over the top of the two piles and paddled it through the messy greasy mélange for an hour and a half, blending up a super-rich mix to be used in spring vegetable planting. Rich compost means disease free, bug free super tasty veggies from now till October.

To top off the day, I moved two huge wheel barrow loads of dry firewood up close to the house for the week's fireplace burn. At 8 p.m. I was done for the day.

Six straight hours of manual labor yesterday.

I worked six straight hours, from 2 to 8 p.m., non-stop, with a generally vigorous activity level on my knee and my brain. You Dear Reader, can evaluate if that is a different state of being for Jim Lindl than he was at on December 5th, only 128 days ago. Remarkable to say the least, I think. Last night my knee was a bit sore, but I was not particularly tired after a big hearty meal. I haven't been able to work like that in several years. Call it Lyme disease, call it chronic fatigue, call it my previous broken spirited condition, call it anything you want . . . but it's gone and the only thing different in my life has been the Teasel tinctures and some high powered vitamins. That's it!

Yesterday was a good day and I'm truly grateful for all the people involved in this incredible journey that began with a visit to Dr. Halverstadt's office in San Luis Obispo, California in mid-September, 2015. That's only 7 months ago. Seven months ago I was a broken spirited man with no understanding why my life had fallen apart. Yes indeed, I'm extremely grateful. To everybody . . . particularly *Mr. Teasel*.

Last night we had 18 mm of soaking hard rain. Good timing for the fertilizer. Today at this keyboard my knee feels pretty darn good. Those x-rays on Tuesday won't lie. They'll be very interesting to evaluate.

June 7th is coming up pretty fast and my Waddington

publishing summit is looming in the ethereal mist of my dreams. I can feel an almost spiritual gravitational pull to launching Mr. Teasel into the public domain. I want to telephone Adolf and tell him of my publishing summit attempt coming up June 7th. He was a "German War Child" and survived the Dresden fire bombings. His uncommon persona of resolve and focus has been an inspiration to me all my life. I want him to know that he made a difference in one person's life . . . for a lifetime. I'm going to call him today.

The German Teasel Family

Wednesday May 4, 2016, 10:41 a.m.

Dear Reader, I've been off the keyboards for 23 days and I can tell the days of writing the Mr. Teasel Story are coming to an end pretty quickly. Maybe another twenty pages . . . tops.

My life has transitioned away from that of a dying dispirited person to a person fully on purpose every day of his life . . . busy, with extensive daily to-do lists that rarely get entirely completed with important tasks needing to be rolled into the next day. We're off to Germany tomorrow for an important 3,500 km road trip to meet the Teasel Family. These are the producers whose Teasel product I took for 82 straight days, beginning December 5th. I had originally hoped to gain a business appointment to meet with them for maybe two to three uninterrupted hours. As it turns out, my wife and I have been invited as their home-stay guests with their family for an entire week! There'll be plenty to report in this journal when we return in 12 days.

Tuesday May 17, 2016, 2:20 p.m.
We've Returned From Germany. Incredible Trip.

In our lifetimes, my wife and I have lived on 3 continents, in

4 countries and experienced day-to-day life in both the Northern and Southern Hemisphere. We've traveled the world, most of it in a non-tourist mode, most of it as serious cultural explorers, seeking insight about different social anomalies not apparent in college text books. Real world everyday life on the street, in people's homes, and in their communities is something that is always on my subconscious radar screen.

I've always been a keen student observing the why and the how that different communities tick and run. I like to analyze why some large groups of people are very socially happy and smile a lot, and some other groups are socially very angry. Thick cultural life on the street level, to me, is one of the ultimate social educational truths far beyond the naïve propaganda of TV sound bites or glib shallow trendy headlines. I've been a lifelong student of the myriad of different social contracts within which people live.

Probably because of my own hardscrabble intersection with some gritty elements of life at an early age, these visceral observations are very important to me. Maybe I'm a keen social observer because I personally experienced repeated cruel injustice and destructive teacher ridicule for stuttering at that Catholic grade school. Who knows. It's just a part of who I am . . . and probably will stay with me till my dying days.

Dear Reader, I can tell you that after an intimate immersion as house guests with three generations of East Germans who have experienced some vast social reorganizations themselves, spanning the total collapse of Germany under crushing Russian armies during WW II, to the grinding Soviet era occupation, to the fall of the Soviet Union in 1990, to the reunification with West Germany, to today's vibrant multicultural evolution of Berlin and hyper-modern living . . . I'm completely humbled by the strength of the human condition to be able to not only get through such extraordinary tough patches of life, but also adapt and thrive and be totally happy and optimistic and thankful for it all. Extraordinary experience for me, inspiring for me, to experience a home-stay with such wonderful hospitable people who have come through so much with so little and opened their home to us with uncommonly warm hospitality to virtual strangers. I wish I was that strong. I wish I was that naturally gracious. They are a model of humanity I want to be more like.

The Future Is Unfolding Right Here & Right Now

Where do I begin writing today . . . ? Or maybe the question should be . . . how do I bring this book to some sort of conclusion?

Is it even possible to bring this book to an end or is this six months of writing and healing and pondering just the beginning of something much bigger? I know the answer and I believe any reader who has followed this journal knows the answer by now. The problem for me is what do I write about in the next few pages to bring this lengthy manuscript to a satisfying and meaningful conclusion for the reader? For the first time in this book I feel like I'm lost for words and have to just wing it and hope for the best in these last few pages. I'll try my best. I've had a zillion interconnected thoughts swimming through my buzzy brain ever since the first day of our home-stay in Germany. I've had a zillion thoughts about things that are happening today that will be interconnected with another zillion things twenty five years from now. By the time we left Berlin, we had gained new fast friends with bold ideas and an earnest desire to do big things together with Teasel. Something bigger than ourselves. I know that others will eventually be involved with the far ranging thoughts we shared over dinner on our last night in Germany. We seven human beings talked in respectful, almost reverent tones, about our plans in the dim candle light well past midnight. We spoke in German, English, Ukrainian, Russian and some French.

We all spoke in discrete bits and pieces of languages that seemed to connect with a particular thought. It was like there were no barriers in front of us. It was like a linguistic table of Babel that dinner evening . . . and we all seemed to know exactly what the thread was of our connection for the future. We were two house guests in a multi-lingual world that night. It was spiritual. The grand patriarch was the center of that spirit.

We talked Teasel production methods, limitations and expansion possibilities with help from other German farmers. We talked about multi-lingual websites, we talked about global outreach, and we talked about their life and ours. Our common intersection that night was our human harmony and our shared vision for introducing the world to healthier possibilities through our joint efforts . . . one person at a time . . . with a goal to leave no stone unturned in the process.

They're coming to France in late July to stay with us to vacation and to further advance our vision for the future of the Foundation and Teasel healing. Possibly we'll be planting some Teasel on our farm someday. Who knows. They've begun reading Mr. Teasel and are in discussions with their son's high school to initiate a student project to translate Mr. Teasel and our new website into German. All of this positive motion was begun during our brief home-stay. Amazing proactive energetic positive people.

Here is the bottom line from our trip: Infected ticks are going to bite more people each year. Lyme disease is not going away. In fact it's spreading and getting worse each year. Specially prepared Teasel tinctures can help alleviate Lyme symptoms as witnessed by these producers over the past nine years and extensively written about by professor Storl, myself and many others.

Our goal is simple but the task is difficult and will take years to accomplish. We want to inform people, worldwide, about what we know and have experienced with Teasel. That's our mission. This book is part of that process. Our Foundation and its website Blog are part of that process.

Because this personal healing journey of mine is evolving and continuing to unfold in unseen ways, I know this book's story does not end here. The book's story and my journey will be continued on the Teasel Foundation website Blog. It's impossible to put to words all that I feel is going to happen in the future.

These 367 pages and now, over 99,000 words, are the opening to a new future for a lot of people who today, May 17, 2016, have no knowledge about Teasel and what's written here. This book is the beginning . . . not the ending.

Concluding Remarks On
The Teasel Foundation Pre-Launch Activity

Saturday May 21, 2016, 11:14 a.m.

Since returning home from Germany another wonderful burst of energy has enveloped this Teasel Foundation in these early budding stages of formation, preparation and launch.

I have long known that the wife of Doctor Blanchard, the Atlas Chiropractor written about in the book, is a native French Canadian speaker and has deep roots in Quebec, Canada. What I didn't know, is that she has been a quiet background reader of the book and has been smitten by Mr. Teasel Fever!

You'll be hearing lots more about her on the English website blog, but especially seeing her work and presence on the French Teasel Foundation website and the French edition of Mr. Teasel! As her time permits, she has volunteered to be the guiding spirit for all the French translation relating to the Foundation website and the book, *Mr. Teasel My Hero*.

This new development gives us a powerful boost to share our holistic healing message, the Teasel Story and the book, with French speakers in both Canada and here in France. Lyme disease is a huge issue all across France and I was wondering how and when we were going to get this book written in French. Unbelievable good luck for our Foundation so early in our development. We haven't even launched yet and we now have both French and German editions of the website, and the book, into serious planning and development. Unbelievable! WOW! English, French and German editions of the book and a fully expressive website in three languages. I have always firmly believed that our important personal visions will manifest if we're just bold enough to think big and believe . . . and have the courage to get into action even if all the details aren't clear.

Like mountaineering . . . even if the weather's sketchy, and the route isn't clearly defined to the summit on a particular technical mountain climb, an earnest mountaineer will take on the challenge believing they have a good chance of success. That's how I feel about this Foundation achieving its objectives. We don't have it all figured out yet, but we know where the summit is and we're definitely on a route to the top!!

Summary Conclusion Of My Healing Journey

Today is exactly 6 months since I began writing this journal on November 21, 2015. Exactly 182 days ago. This is a good time to summarize and wrap up.

When I began the opening thoughts back then, I clearly stated I had two overarching objectives: Firstly, I wanted to beat my Lyme disease symptoms with a non-pharmaceutical approach . . . a holistic approach. It worked out in triple full house spades. I'm a totally different person today than 182 days ago.

Secondly, I wanted to avoid imminent knee surgery and eventually grow new knee cartilage. It's been a disappointment to not get any new cartilage started yet. I'm hopeful that with more and different nutrification and different combinations of phyto-therapy I'll eventually get something happening in the next 12 months. For now I'm extremely thankful that I can at least function on that bum knee, at least partially. The pain is only present when I walk on hard pavement and over exert with too much walking. I found my limits in Berlin on hard sidewalks. The following new set of x-rays tells the entire story. My right knee is still bone on bone contact and not at all good.

My next move, if the natural cartilage regeneration does not eventually work out, is to head to Denver and see the Regenexx folks for stem cell treatment. I can't stress enough, that anybody who thinks they need a hip replacement, knee replacement or spinal fusion, should seriously consider reading all the Regenexx links in this e-Book. Go to the Regenexx blog archives and dig through the 2,000+ articles. Search by subject matter, and get educated about the dangers and pitfalls of conventional orthopedic surgery and possibilities of stem cell treatment. Please read everything before you go under the knife. Get educated.

I could request an appointment with my wonderful French Orthopedic Surgeon tomorrow and probably get scheduled for a knee replacement very soon, but I won't succumb to that temptation. The entire procedure and healing program, no matter how complicated and involved, is 100% covered by insurance. The doctors and medical systems here in France are some of the best in the world. Why won't I go this route? Dear Reader, read about the life expectancy of a TKR . . . 15 years max! Then what? Another total double bone amputation/joint removal and joint replacement again at age 79? Think about that challenge to a person at age 79. No thank you. I'm a future thinker and planner who lives in the reality of today.

Read about the infected blood poisoning and long term complications due to foreign particle contamination from an artificial joint. Not good data over the past 20 years. Big immune system troubles can arise from that constant deposition of foreign particles introduced into the blood every day for the rest of a person's life. These are the realities and the outcomes if everything goes well and there's no rejection and complication. A knee replacement can go downhill pretty fast if there are complications with such a massively disruptive surgery.

I ask myself today . . . what did people do 50 years ago before these massive orthopedic interventions were available? Cut off their leg and put a prosthetic on the stump I suppose.

I can do that. Look at all the war veterans in far worse shape than me. Because of all I've learned and the options available with holistic healing and/or stem cell treatment . . . surgery has been postponed and will remain off the table in my thinking . . . forever.

I choose to limp with limited mobility for the foreseeable future and will continue to manage and to improve my knee condition holistically . . . forever.

That's my decision. Readers of The Teasel Foundation blog can get periodic updates as to the how and the what I'm currently doing towards that goal.

As far as I'm concerned, the Lyme symptoms are dead, buried and just an interesting foot note in Jim Lindl's past history. I've been careful to write about my "Lyme symptoms" not my 'Lyme disease." And here is the reason: After I got bitten by that tick 8 years ago, the first blood test, the one listed first in this book, indicated Lyme negative but did suggest a second test was appropriate if Lyme like symptoms continued. Well . . . the symptoms did continue and got worse, but I never did a second test until 7 years later when I couldn't think clearly or walk unassisted. That was last Fall, 2015. That second test indicated essentially the same result as the first one, but it further stated, that even though my Lyme antibody count was not strongly indicating Lyme bacteria, I may very well have Lyme disease anyhow. That type of change in test language indicates to me they are pretty unsure of the validity of the current state of Lyme bacteria testing.

My internet research seems to confirm this thinking. In other words, those two tests may be totally useless to definitively indicate if Lyme bacteria are present or not. Therefore, I use the term, "Lyme symptoms" throughout the book because I can't be certain if I ever had "Lyme disease" from those two test results. Nor does anybody else, but . . . my surgeon was suspicious enough of my symptoms that he had me slated to go through some further advanced Lyme testing before knee surgery would be considered.

The third and final Lyme test from a few weeks ago confirms my bias that the current state of Lyme testing is deficient and not trustworthy. This latest Lyme test indicates that absolutely nothing has changed in the three blood tests over the past eight years. **Nothing had changed according to the blood tests!**

Okay, enough of high tech medical analysis for me. I have to revert back to the Jim Lindl of old, the no BS common sense practical thinking timber cutter of old.

I say if it looks like a duck, quacks like a duck, walks like a duck and tastes like a duck dinner on the dining room table . . . then it must be a duck! That's the best way I can summarize what I think about my "Lyme symptoms" and these three nebulous tests that the French medical community is not even sure about. Call my condition whatever you want, my Lyme duck doesn't quack anymore! Zero symptoms. No quacking! I'm happy!

You Dear Reader need to draw your own conclusions from the evidence of this journal but here is the third blood test taken a month ago that says that maybe I have Lyme disease and maybe I don't but a retest in 30 days is a good idea!! They have been saying that same thing for the past eight years! If I had relied on those tests exclusively for the past 8 years and not consulted with Dr. Halverstadt about my puzzling and debilitating condition, I'd still be a complete mess to this very day. I'll consider revisiting that past someday if my "ocular lightning flashes" reappear, or the chronic fatigue returns and puts me down every day at 4 p.m. or my memory starts to go haywire again. But until then, I consider my past encounter with a tick in the middle of French Lyme disease country . . .

"Case Closed." Thank You MR.TEASEL, You Are My Hero.

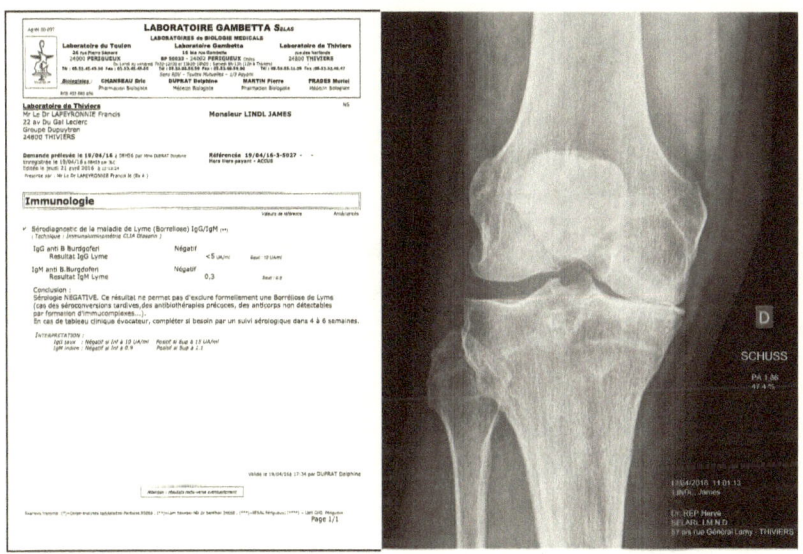

My Blood Work
April 19, 2016
© 2016 Jim Lindl

My Right Knee X-Ray
April 12, 2016
© 2016 Jim Lindl

Epilogue

The book and the website did not get launched on June 7th as originally planned. We forfeited three months of valuable time because we redirected our "Waddington summit approach" in midstream towards a bigger vision, an even taller summit objective that unexpectedly came into clear full view in the past three months.

Mountaineering surprises can often dictate route changes. Optimal business plan execution can also require mid-course corrections. Once we could clearly see that a German and French language version of Mr. Teasel was going to happen, we knew it was time to broaden our web design thinking, international in scope, right from the launch. It became apparent this was the correct decision.

However, I don't believe we actually lost any of our publishing momentum in the longer term picture because we gained a much bigger vision and gained a multi-lingual global reach early in the process that will ultimately lead to many more Lyme affected people much quicker, worldwide.

I have purposely not included a final review of any products I took during this book writing and healing journey over the past six months, and not because those products are unimportant. Quite the contrary. I have not written anything more about specific products in my daily regime because an entire book could be written about the eleven different nutritional products I experimented with for optimal nutrification. Particularly the products for my knee cartilage repair. Plus, there were seven phyto-therapy products, in addition to the teasel, that I have experimented with over the course of the past six months. Again, mainly for my knee troubles. A person dealing strictly with Lyme symptoms certainly doesn't need to take everything I have incorporated into my knee healing protocols. For Lyme, if a person simply gets the Teasel Tick Kit, the Bee Extract Killer Biotics, some effective nutrification vitamins, and Wolf Storl's book they will be on their way. I have very high expectations for my knee recovery and I'm dealing with it accordingly. The website blog will be the arena to follow that knee healing progress.

My overarching goal in this book has evolved into a passion to expose the reader to the possibilities of herbal and nutritional therapy through my story. I'll leave the reader to their own exploration of products, but I highly recommend that a chat with CK is an excellent first step in that direction. She provided me with many of the basic nutritional product ideas and the healing logic behind them. She also facilitated a very efficient purchase process and door to door delivery service direct to me in France. She can do the same for you. She's a trustee and director of the Foundation but also works with us in a supportive fundraising role, not a conflicted role, with her nutritional business. That relationship is explained on the Mr. Teasel website within the fundraising discussion.

I personally will continue reaching out to teasel producers, herbalists and Lyme educators, worldwide, for their help in supplying superior quality teasel tinctures and their expert knowledge for our Foundation website. I have found one excellent teasel producer that helped me and I will continue looking for more. I suspect we'll need all the producers we can find as this book gains a wide readership. CK will know who these producers are and how to reach them.

Tens upon tens of thousands of new Lyme cases each year is a lot of potential teasel tincture demand which I don't believe the producers can fully accommodate today. Maybe one day The Teasel Foundation itself will have its own experiential phyto-therapy production and educational farm and a modern tincture research and production center influenced by the Old World Traditions.

I'm Hopeful

I'm hopeful for the future about a lot of things after writing this book and forming the Teasel Foundation. Together, with your help spreading the message of this book and introducing people to our website . . . maybe just maybe… with your voice and mine, we can accomplish some good things together. Thank you for reading this lengthy story. I hope it helps you or it helps somebody you know with their Lyme disease or their Lyme disease symptoms.

Jim Lindl
Dordogne, France
June 1st, 2016

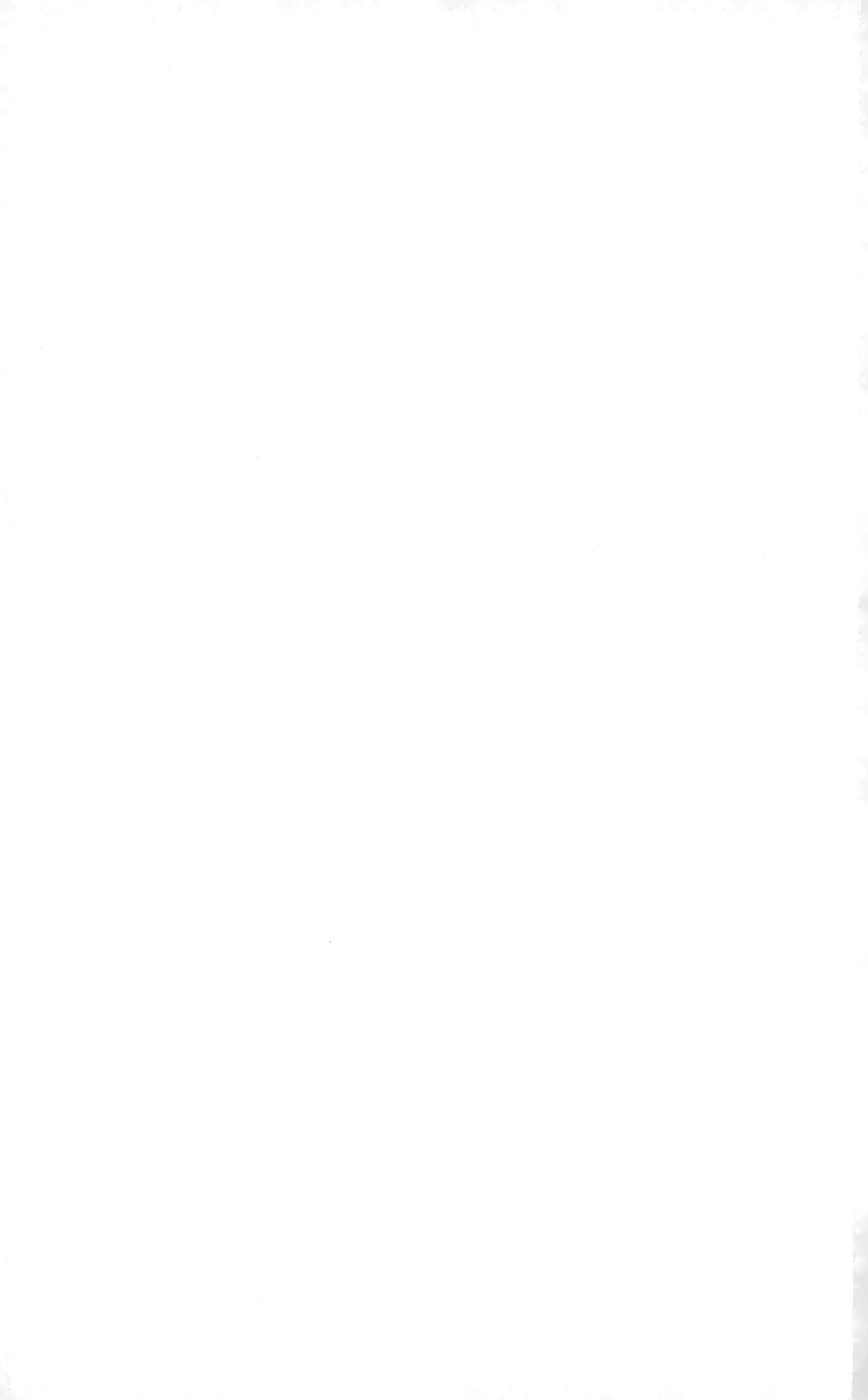

www.ingramcontent.com/pod-product-compliance
Lightning Source LLC
Chambersburg PA
CBHW022046160426
43198CB00008B/143